Dedication

To my beloved Ruth and the scores of people who played roles
in the progressive struggles of my lifetime and to those
brave enough to take the struggles forward.

Acknowledgements

First and foremost to Steve Fiffer for his abiding partnership in the development of this book—endless hours of interviews, reviewing of newspaper articles, and ultimately writing the book. Steve had the constant belief that my story was worth telling and might actually mean something in the forward movement of history.

Kevin Leonard and the archives department at Northwestern University where my papers are kept were so supportive of this project and provided all of my papers to Steve.

Mardge Cohen, Gordy Schiff, Peter Orris, Claudia Fegan, Lon Berkeley, Jack Raba, Linda Murray for their close review and commenting on various chapters of this book.

This book chronicles nearly a century of my life and I am indebted to the thousands of people I have worked with at Cook County Hospital, at Health and Medicine Policy Research Group, at Physicians for a National Health Program (PNHP), at WBEZ (Chicage Public Radio), in private practice, in labor unions, activists of many stripes, my patients, and so many more. You have all taught me so much over these years.

Special thanks to Mark Almberg and Ida Hellander of PNHP for their help in writing chapter 13 about PNHP and the single-payer movement.

Thanks to the board of HMPRG for pushing me to write this book and for helping underwrite the cost of producing it. Many thanks to Health and Medicine's Office Manager Ann Duffy for transcribing the dozens of tapes of Steve Fiffer interviewing me. Special thanks to board member Rachel Reichlin for her close review and prompting of stories to fill in many chapters, and to

Executive Director Margie Schaps for endless hours of reviewing chapter drafts, coaxing stories out of me, and gently (and sometimes not so gently) pushing me to complete this project. Without Margie I think it is safe to say this book might never have been completed.

And finally to my children, stepchildren, their spouses and their children for their constant support during this project.

Prologue

When you get to be my age, there's no shortage of stories to tell about things you've done, people you've met, and places you've been. Whether those stories are interesting enough to fill a book is for you, the reader, to decide. Remembering all these stories and presenting them accurately is another matter. Fortunately in my case there is quite a paper trail. Newspapers have covered many of the events that have highlighted my life—the Freedom Summer in Mississippi, the march for voting rights in Selma, Dr. Martin Luther King's efforts to desegregate Chicago, the police riots associated with the 1968 Democratic Convention, the trial of the Chicago Eight, the travails of Cook County Hospital, the fight for a single-payer health care system, and my stance toward "Obamacare." What the newspapers haven't covered can be found in some of my papers and correspondence from the wonderful organizations with which I have been associated like the Medical Committee for Human Rights, Health and Medicine Policy Research Group, and Physicians for a National Health Program. Another organization also kept an almost daily diary of my activities during the 1960s and 1970s, the Federal Bureau of Investigation. Thanks, guys!

Another function of getting to be my age is that family, friends, and colleagues feel obliged to commemorate birthdays and other milestones on a regular basis. It was at one of these events not too long ago that Gordy Schiff, a longtime friend from my Cook County Hospital days, reminded me and a rather large audience of a story I had forgotten. At a conference on health care chaired by the late U.S. Senator Paul Wellstone, attendees were invited to ask questions. I rose, and as Gordy tells it, I went into a lengthy dissertation about all the ills of society: poverty, racism, and, of course, inadequate health care. Several times during the course of my oration, the moderator asked me what my question was. I ignored him and kept speaking. After several minutes, the exasperated chair finally put his foot down. "Dr. Young," he said. "What is your question?" I paused for a moment, then said, "Am I not right?"

I've fought a lot of battles over the years. I've won some and lost many. Sometimes I've been willing to compromise, and many times I haven't. I've built bridges and burned bridges. Have I been right? Read on and decide for yourself.

—Quentin Young, M.D.
September 1, 2013

One

If not for my Aunt Dora, the bootlegger, this book might never have been written. It's fair to say that much of whatever notoriety I have derives from my longtime association with Cook County Hospital in Chicago. That association began in the late 1940s when I was an intern and resident. But it was my ten years there as chairman of medicine from 1972 to 1982 that were chock full of headlines about palace intrigue and, fortunately, some historic breakthroughs in the field of public health.

I almost didn't get that job. No job, no book (or at least not nearly as interesting a story). That's where Dora comes in.

A little history: from its earliest days, County (now called John H. Stroger Jr. Hospital of Cook County) was not only one of the finest public hospitals in America, it was also a jewel in the crown of Chicago's Democratic Machine. County's administrator served at the pleasure of the pols. Personnel and hospital purchasing decisions were controlled by the local bosses.

Owing their jobs at the hospital to the Machine, workers joined the patronage army that perpetuated the power of the powers that be, including Richard J. Daley, who served as mayor of Chicago and chairman of the Cook County Democratic Central Committee from the mid-1950s until his death in 1976. Vendors paid further tribute in return for lucrative contracts. Beds were filled, and nests were feathered.

In 1969, a Republican governor, Richard Ogilvie, persuaded the Illinois Legislature to put control of the hospital in the hands of an independent citizens commission instead of the County Board of Commissioners. This welcome move didn't completely cure the chronic corruption, but it did reduce the Machine's influence.

Three years later, the commission approached me about becoming chairman of medicine, the largest department in the hospital. Having locked horns with Mayor Daley on previous occasions, including the 1968 convention, I would not have been on the Machine's short list in the "good old days." Indeed, even during this era of reform, I wasn't a shoo-in with the new commission. Believe it or not, some of those who interviewed me were unhappy that I was planning to join a Medical Committee for Human Rights (MCHR) contingent taking medical supplies to a country *non grata* shortly before I was to begin at County.

"I can only stay for an hour," I told my examiners. "I have a plane to catch."

"Where are you going?"

"North Vietnam."

Said one outraged member of the commission: "You'll get this job over my dead body."

"Deal!" I responded, and I headed to the airport.

Enter Dr. Samuel Hoffman. A holdover from the Daley days, he still held considerable sway as director of the County-affiliated Hektoen Institute, which funded clinical research projects. I suspect he was the Machine's overseer, making sure reform did not take up permanent residence before the old guard could regain control of their political plum (which would indeed happen).

I didn't expect Hoffman to be in my corner. Then we started playing Jewish geography. It turned out that in his youth he had known and liked Aunt Dora, a formidable presence on the city's West Side thanks to both personality and Prohibition. Blood being even thicker than politics, I suddenly had a new friend in Hoffman. I got the job.

Dora and my father Abe were two of fourteen siblings in the Lipshitz family. Seven of the children did not survive childhood in Russia. The mother of the children, my grandmother, also died in the Old Country. The survivors emigrated to the United States at the end of the 19th century. When the Lipshitzes arrived at Ellis Island, the story goes, officials instructed them to pull out an American name from a hat. Annette, my Uncle Bob's stepdaughter, drew the name "Young."

The Youngs settled on New York City's Lower East Side before dispersing. By the time I was born in 1923, my father had

2

moved to Chicago to join his brother-in-law Charles Greenhauf in business. They were contractors, making a middle-class living remodeling apartments and building garages. We lived in a modest house on the city's South Side, less than half a mile west of the University of Chicago. Although a synagogue sat across the street, our neighborhood was primarily Catholic.

My mother Sarah's people had come to the U.S. from Lithuania. Her father had settled in, of all places, Oxford, North Carolina, a town of a few thousand people, twenty-five miles southwest of Durham. He started out as a peddler. Eventually he quit the road, opened up a four-story general store, and became a prominent member of the community.

Before moving to Chicago, my father had earned a degree in pharmacology from Fordham University. He had hoped to go on to medical school, but couldn't afford it. So he became a salesman, traveling much of the Eastern seaboard selling jewelry. He'd met my mother in Oxford on one of his trips. They married in 1922, when she was 19 and he was about 25.

Quentin, I realize, is hardly the quintessential Jewish name. The story goes that my mother wanted to name her first born after Teddy Roosevelt's youngest son. Quentin Roosevelt was a courageous World War I flyer killed over France at age 20 in 1917. His death struck a chord with the nation, including then 14-year-old Sarah Wolf.

Jewish tradition mandates naming the first-born son after a deceased relative. There were no Quentins in the old (or new) country, or, for that matter, relatives whose name began with Q. Apparently, however, there had been an Uncle Chloina. Close enough. My mother wrote to the authoritative Jewish newspaper, *The Forward*, to ask if Quentin was a permissible substitute for Chloina. The paper, presumably after consulting a scholar or two, bestowed its blessing. QED.

My mother and I spent several summers in Oxford. I can honestly say I was Oxford-educated because we stayed with my mother's parents for an entire year when I was six or seven and I went to the local one-room schoolhouse that served kids from kindergarten through eighth grade. Of course the school was segregated, as was most everything in the South in those days (not that Chicago and the North were much better). My grandfather's store welcomed blacks—as long as they did not try on any clothes.

There weren't a lot of Jewish families in my grandparents' neighborhood. I played with Gorham Webb, an older kid from down the street; he was the younger brother of the local congressman. Fast forward about fifteen years. Gorham was a prisoner of war, captured by the Japanese in the Philippines early in World War II. When he finally returned home, Oxford held a parade in his honor. My grandmother saw him and they embraced. When asked about their reunion, she said, *"This is the first time I've ever kissed a goy."* (Goy is the Yiddish word for Gentile. I picked up quite a bit of Yiddish at home, including the three degrees of *meshugana,* or crazy person: first degree is *meshuga*, the second degree is *takka meshuga*, or really crazy, and then *ganze meshuga*, entirely crazy.)

As a city boy, I was curious to see one of the local tobacco farms. My grandfather indulged me, taking me to a farm outside Durham. There we saw workers in the field pulling and bundling leaves; we saw where the tobacco was cured; and we saw machines cutting long strands into cigarette-sized sticks. In my youthful zeal, I actually lit one of the strands and took a few puffs... and got quite sick. (Unfortunately this early lesson in the negative effects of tobacco did not prevent me from smoking when I got to college.)

While my memory of the cigarette-making process is hazy, I still remember what stirred me most on that visit more than eighty years ago: watching the tobacco field workers. They were all black—almost exclusively older women and children my age, whom I learned were kept out of their segregated schools until the season ended later in the fall. Their clothes were ragged and torn.

I was too young to have a political orientation, but I could sense that their worth to their farmer-bosses depended on how much they could pick. The women and children didn't lollygag. They looked tired, but worked fast.

Did I sense a difference between the South and the North? Not entirely. Looking back, I realize that as segregated as Chicago

4

was in the 1930s, the racial hierarchy was not quite as woven into the fabric of life. In North Carolina, the blacks just seemed to know they could not enter a drugstore or restaurant and sit down and order. They knew, too, that they must avoid touching merchandise in the white-owned stores. Black kids, I know now, were told from infancy, "You don't go here. You don't talk (or even whistle) there." Similarly, an innocent white kid who might have the inclination to play with black kids learned his own set of rules; socializing with the "colored" was taboo.

Life on Chicago's South Side was not nearly as exotic as it was in the South. I led a pretty normal, quiet life with my sister Tina, four years my junior. As I was the oldest and a boy and as she was saddled with a harelip, I was doted upon. Given a great deal of freedom, I played with our neighbors, went to the movies or live vaudeville shows on Saturday mornings, passed the holidays at Aunt Dora's, and studied for my bar mitzvah. For a while, I thought I wanted to be a rabbi.

That changed as I approached my coming of age at thirteen and was politicized. Fascism was growing around the world and lefties like me felt it was an immediate menace. The friends I made when I was thirteen were not Jewish. We connected more politically, and the desire to become a rabbi waned.

I read a lot. Edgar Rice Burroughs' *Tarzan* series was my favorite. I was no whiz kid, but the teachers at my public school did bump me up two grades—not an unusual phenomenon back then.

If there was one activity that separated me from my peers, it was the Jack and Jill Players, a well-known children's acting troupe that performed onstage and on the radio. These days when I meet people they often tell me they remember me from the radio. I know they are talking about my association over the last quarter-century with the Chicago public radio station WBEZ, where I hosted one show and appeared frequently on others. These new friends have no idea that as a kid of about twelve or thirteen, I appeared on such national radio broadcasts as "Jack Armstrong, All American Boy" and "Little Orphan Annie," each of which launched from Chicago in the early 1930s. I also played the murderous Bill Sykes in a long-forgotten stage version of Dickens'

Oliver Twist. An acting stretch if ever there was one, though I've probably employed my favorite line from the play many times over the years under different circumstances: "I ain't afraid of you, Sykes."

My mother was no Mama Rose, but she was the driving force behind my thespian efforts. Impressed by my ability to tell a joke and do dialects, she placed me with the Players. I would ride the el downtown for auditions, rehearsals, and performances. The pay was never great, but I did learn to be at ease speaking to large audiences. (I've been asked if my friend, the late, great Studs Terkel, was also a member of the Players as a youngster. My answer: Studs was never a youngster.)

Sometimes my acting interfered with school. I thought my balancing act was going pretty well until a science teacher at Hyde Park High School took me aside and said, "If you miss one more class, I'm going to flunk you." And so the curtain came down on that brief career.

By the time I entered high school in 1936, we had moved to a house at 68th and Cornell, a little more than a mile south of the University of Chicago. I rode my Schwinn to school. That may sound Norman Rockwell-innocent, but the times were anything but. The country was in the middle of the Great Depression. Unemployment was rampant. There was union-management conflict, too.

Abroad, Hitler was in control of Germany. Mussolini's Italy had invaded Ethiopia. The Spanish Civil War had just begun. I followed these events closely and cared deeply about those under the fists of the Fascists.

Where did this social and political conscience come from? I don't know. My parents were New Deal Democrats. Upon occasion, they invited African Americans to dinner. But Abe and Sarah were not the least bit radical. They did not condone my infatuation with the left, but by the time I was a teen they had given up on trying to control me.

My political awareness and outrage grew even stronger when I joined the American Student Union at Hyde Park High. ASU had been formed in 1935 by folks who considered themselves Communists or Socialists or Progressives. The group's anti-Nazi, pro-Spanish-Republican stance drew me in. This was a college-centered movement, but there were about a half dozen active chapters at high schools in the Chicago area. We didn't have a room or a faculty adviser for our 150 members at the high school, but students from the nearby University of Chicago helped us organize a council that brought in speakers and lobbied for progressive causes at home and overseas.

Over the years, those with whom I've done battle, including the House Un-American Activities Committee (HUAC), have often pointed to my ASU membership as evidence that I was a Commie. (More recently some on the right have gone a step further, saying that those who associated with the ASU-affiliated Quentin Young must themselves be dangerous radicals. In 2008, for example, Barack Obama was attacked for his friendship with me.) Truth be told, I've never been one for labels, and at age fourteen or fifteen, I really wasn't aware of who was what. I was oblivious to the fact that there was a split between ASU's Communists and Socialists that would eventually lead to a divorce.

My conscience was also nurtured by a remarkable history teacher at the high school, Walter Hipple. A real 1920s radical who challenged us to make a difference, he often invited students to his home for dinner and political conversation. My lifelong friend Bernice Weissbourd, then Bernice Targ, remembers that Mr. Hipple frequently lamented that we were all going to end up in the mainstream instead of agitating for change. (That was one thing he got wrong: Bernice has been a leader in progressive causes for over sixty years. She is perhaps best known for founding Family Focus, a wonderful organization that promotes the well-being of children from birth by supporting and strengthening their families in and with their communities.)

While the world may forever associate Chicago with the St. Valentine's Day Massacre of 1929, I was shaped by the Memorial Day Massacre of 1937. In the former, seven rival gang members were gunned down in a Lincoln Park garage by mobsters associated with Al Capone. Two of the shooters dressed as policemen. In the latter, real Chicago policemen gunned down ten unarmed demonstrators near the Republic Steel Mill on Chicago's South Side. Another thirty people were injured.

The demonstrators had gathered to march in support of what was called the "Little Steel Strike." After smaller steel manufacturers had refused to agree to the union contract approved by the larger U.S. Steel, the Steelworkers Organizing Committee of the Congress of Industrial Organizations had called the strike. Blocked from their course by the Chicago police, the peaceful marchers threw a tree branch at the cops. In response, Chicago's finest opened fire. Later, a coroner's jury would, shamefully, term the shootings "justifiable homicide." The incident, a turning point in the organization of steelworkers, left a stain on the city, a monument at the site, and an indelible impression on me at thirteen.

I was not at the demonstration, but I did attend a large rally downtown at Orchestra Hall in the aftermath. There, a young lawyer named Leon "Len" Despres eloquently described what had happened. He would go on to great things in Chicago, representing the 5th Ward (which included Hyde Park) as an alderman from 1955 to 1975. He was long the conscience of the City Council and often the lone "nay" when Mayor Daley pushed through legislation that benefited his cronies at the expense of the disenfranchised. He fought tirelessly for racial equality in everything from housing to city hiring. On more than one occasion, the mayor ordered Len's microphone shut off in the middle of an impassioned plea for fairness or indignant condemnation of the Machine.

Len was a fascinating guy. In the 1930s, he had been the guest of Leon Trotsky at the revolutionary Marxist's Mexican villa. (If they were not fellow travelers, they were at least fellow Leons.) Also in Mexico, he and his wife Marian had befriended the famed artist Frida Kahlo and her husband, the equally renowned Diego Rivera. While Rivera painted a portrait of Marian, Len took Ms. Kahlo to the cinema.

Years after the memorable speech at Orchestra Hall, Len and I became friends and political allies. Eventually I became his doctor. (I'd like to take credit for the fact that he lived until he was 101. In truth, however, I think he was blessed with good genes and kept himself alive by maintaining his law practice until the very end.)

I don't want to give the impression that righting the world's wrongs was the only thing on my teenage mind. While I wasn't into the party scene like some of my high school classmates, I thought a lot about girls. This explains why dating as well as politics was on the list of things I hoped to discuss when I made an appointment in the spring of 1940 with Sid Lipshire, the elected head of the University of Chicago's ASU chapter.

I had just graduated from high school and would be entering the U. of C. in the fall. Where else would a leftward-leaning Hyde Parker go? I'd never met Sid, but I figured he could enlighten me on the campus political scene and give me some pointers on girls.

We met on campus in his office. These were tough times for ASU. Many members from across the country, including the U. of C., had gone to fight in the Spanish Civil War. Some had been killed. At the same time, the organization was going through an identity crisis. ASU was fiercely leftist. Now, however, some of those world leaders whom we had touted were disappointing us. In August 1939, the Soviet Union's Josef Stalin had entered into a non-aggression pact with the hated Hitler. Ouch.

Sid and I began by discussing the headache that was known as the Hitler-Stalin Pact. We then lamented the imperialistic policies of France and Britain and for that matter the U.S. This was standard ASU conversation, and we were on the same page, although he was far more knowledgeable.

I'd entered the meeting in awe of this college guy four years my senior who was running a 500-member organization. But he quickly put me at ease. He was a bright, committed, middle-class Jewish kid from the East Coast.

Feeling comfortable, I turned the talk to what I think I described as "the state of arrangements between boys and girls." I explained that those arrangements seemed to consist of necking parties with lights out and parents in the next room. I wanted something better than such "structured oppression" of women and refused to indulge, I told him.

Sid did not provide the type of guidance I was expecting. Instead, he asked, "What do you think of Jessie Polacheck?"

Hmm. I knew Jessie, a fellow ASU member who was my age, but a year behind me at Hyde Park High because of my promotions. We saw each other every day. But I hadn't given any thought at all to her in the way Sid seemed to be suggesting I should—romantically. In fact, I'd been somewhat unkind to her, dismissive.

Sid drew a great image of a left-wing approach to a personal situation and how we would look to the next generation. Liberated. A bunch of malarkey like that. So I was very taken with what he had to say.

I suddenly looked with different eyes upon Miss Polacheck. Wearing a babushka (headscarf) and no make-up, she had seemed a bit comical to me. Sid explained that this liberated look was the wave of the future.

Jessie lived a stone's throw from the ASU office on 57th Street between Blackstone and Dorchester. When I left my meeting with Sid, I ran to her house. She was home with a bad cold, but, as I recall, *she* thought there was something wrong with *me*. I hadn't come to profess my love—I was there as a colleague—but I was friendly. In the past, I'd treated her somewhere between ridicule and contempt. (And yet, I later learned, she'd had a crush on me. Go figure.)

Over the days and weeks ahead, we bonded, became close friends, dated, and talked about the future. In the fall I was off to college and she was back to high school, but we remained a couple. Keep reading and you can follow our trials and tribulations over the years that followed.

The University of Chicago lived up to my expectations. When I entered in 1940, Robert Maynard Hutchins was the president. He was famous for numerous reforms including eliminating football, building a curriculum around the Great Books, and instituting comprehensive year-end examinations. "It must be remembered that the purpose of education is not to fill the minds of students with facts... but to teach them to think," he explained. (He's also remembered for a quotation that still makes me chuckle, although I could never tell it to a patient: "Whenever I feel the need to exercise, I lie down until it goes away.")

I would have been perfectly content to spend the next four years in my beloved Hyde Park, studying the liberal arts, preparing for a career in medicine, agitating for justice in the U.S. and Europe, and courting Jessie. But everything changed on December 7, 1941.

Two

Don't tell anyone, but I never graduated from college.

I certainly entered the University of Chicago in 1940 with every intention of doing so. And once there, I loved the curriculum instituted by President Hutchins. Under the "Chicago Plan," all students in the college took two-year courses in the humanities; the natural sciences; the social sciences; and reading, writing, and criticism. We also took a one-year course in philosophy and two departmental electives and had to demonstrate our competency in math and a foreign language. Although we had traditional assignments, little, if anything, was mandatory. Our entire grade was based on a six-hour examination at the end of the nine-month school year. How utopian!

Sometime during my first or second year, I decided that I wanted to be a doctor. "Why?" you ask. Because medicine was the profession most in keeping with my system of beliefs. It was a livelihood that offered the opportunity to do good (not that every doctor takes up the offer). Yes, it was a relatively tough academic ride, but if you could make it to the end and get your license, you could earn a comfortable living. And, if you so chose, you could go to work every day and be a decent, caring, supportive person practicing your profession.

Although my father had seen his dreams of being a doctor dashed for financial reasons, he didn't push me to make this career choice. Nor did I have any role models in the medical community. My interaction with doctors up to this point was blessedly uneventful. Except for my sister's harelip, no one in our family had suffered any serious maladies. The biggest medical event in my life had been the removal of my tonsils.

A few words about doctors and the practice of medicine in those days. Doctors were almost all general practitioners; specialization was just beginning and was reserved for complex, difficult cases when available. The doctors were mostly in the neighborhoods as opposed to downtown office buildings. There were no antibiotics. If you were sick, the doctor might give you an aspirin and tell you to rest for a few days. People didn't have the same cost burden of disease, because access to expensive curative methods was in the future.

The introduction of antibiotics and anesthesia represented a complete transformation of the way medicine was practiced. Further expansion of pharmaceuticals, and the advancement of medicine with a focus on curative treatment created a new approach to medical care.

Penicillin and sulfa drugs were just discovered in the mid-1940s. Only in the latter half of the 20th century did the specialty of anesthesia come to fruition. The first successful removal of a lung was 1938, at a time when there were really no antibiotics. This was the beginning of surgery as a modality for treatment of serious disease.

On the occasions that anyone in our family needed medical care in the 1920s and '30s, my parents paid cash. I think a visit to the doctor in those days cost about three dollars. We didn't have health insurance, nor did our friends. My father didn't provide health benefits to his employees.

So how did folks pay? Those who couldn't pay often got a reduced bill. Others would pay off the debt over the years or even barter goods or services in exchange for treatment.

As the capacity to do high cost surgical procedures increased, so did the need for insurance. In effect, the insurance system was developing at the same time as the advancement of surgical and medical management. Implementation began through the unions in the big industries like steel, meatpacking, and auto. It was *not* universal. A large portion of the population had job-related insurance, but a bigger proportion did not have insurance, even though they worked.

At U. of C., all students were covered for medical care. But there was a dual system for those needing hospitalization: white students were admitted to the U. of C. hospital, but black students were sent to Provident Hospital, a dilapidated hospital on the other side of Washington Park that the university gave to the black community in 1925.

(Jumping ahead a bit to provide some perspective: For the year 1950, the total cost of the American health system was $22 billion. In 2011, the cost of the health system was $2.7 trillion—20 percent of the entire gross domestic product. This reflects the transformation of how medicine was practiced.)

Despite its liberal arts orientation, the University of Chicago Plan was structured so that a student could take what amounted to a pre-med curriculum. This I did. In retrospect I think this was a wonderful educational experience that served me the rest of my life. The Plan gave me a much broader view of what there is to know and what the controversies were, where there were controversies. It's fair to say that my orientations towards local and international issues were developed at this time. To this day, I rely on the skills implied by that education.

During the 1930s and 1940s, many tagged the U. of C. as a "leftist" school. Maybe the fact that the curriculum was progressive and encouraged free-thinking led outsiders to conclude that the university was a hotbed of radicalism. I'd say "warm" is a better description than hot. Certainly, there was a left presence on the campus; we were serious about social issues. But the left was present on campuses across the country. After all, we were still in the Great Depression at home and on the brink of World War II.

As a member of the American Student Union and several ad hoc groups including the American League for Peace and Democracy, I spent much of my time as I do now—in meetings. And just as I complain now that we have more meetings than necessary, so I complained then. In addition to picking up ideas, here's where I picked up my smoking habit, which lasted from age sixteen to thirty-two. (My logic at the time and even now was that I had to learn to smoke because I was inhaling so much smoke from others in the room. This is a poor joke… and even poorer excuse.)

Many people assume that the focus of campus activism was

15

to promote communism. But in my case, and the case of most of my fellow students, we were much more anti-Nazi than pro-Russian. We came not to praise Stalin, but to bury Hitler and Mussolini. We watched with anger and horror as Germany and Russia invaded and conquered Poland and divided the country between themselves. We watched Hitler wage war across Europe in 1940. And we shook our heads and fists when Germany broke its pact with Stalin and invaded Russia in June of 1941. We agitated for U.S. intervention, taking issue with the isolationists who thought we should keep our nose and our troops out of Europe.

Until December 7, 1941, our eyes were less focused on Asia, including the Japanese invasion of China in 1937. But then Pearl Harbor was attacked. I was in downtown Chicago on my way to give a speech—I don't remember the subject or exact locale—when I heard the news that Japan had launched the surprise assault on our naval base in Hawaii. The speech was cancelled, and I returned to Hyde Park, anxious to learn all I could. Compared to today, news traveled at a snail's pace, so it took a few days to learn the extent of the attack. The casualties were staggering: over 2,400 Americans killed and some 1,300 wounded.

President Roosevelt declared war on Japan on December 8. Three days later, in support of their ally Japan, Germany and Italy declared war on the U.S. Many Americans immediately enlisted in the armed forces. Still only seventeen years old, I was too young to enlist; you had to be at least eighteen to sign up or be drafted.

Truth be told, I wasn't ready to go fight. Over the next year, however, as the evil of the axis came into sharper focus, I became passionate about going to war, almost obsessed with the idea of fighting the Nazis. By 1943, when I was nineteen, it was clear that sometime over the next year I would be drafted. As I was pre-med, I would probably have been able to secure a student deferment. But I didn't want to defer defeating Hitler. In March of 1943, I enlisted in the Army.

As a "voluntary inductee," I was supposed to be able to choose my branch of service. Knowing that my nearsightedness would keep me out of my first choice, the infantry, I indicated my preference for the next most lethal branch, artillery. But I quickly learned that you surrender preferences and prerogatives when you enter the Army. You do what they want you to do.

They wanted me to be in the medical department. That made sense. I did have three years of pre-med under my belt. Still, after going through the standard battery of physical and mental exams, I suggested to a sergeant that having voluntarily enlisted I should be allowed to join the artillery. "Shut up and get in line," he told me. And so I became aware of what real power is—and even more aware that I had none.

I entered the Army as a skinny, pack-a-day smoker, who was the poster boy for the Robert Maynard Hutchins School of Exercise Abstinence. In three months I came a long way. Initially, I had trouble walking one mile with a pack on my back. By the end, I could do a 25-mile march, carrying a full pack.

A little nomenclature: The medical corps was comprised of doctors. The medical department was comprised of enlisted men like me of all ages. Most were not pre-med students. We were trained to be medics—to go onto the battlefield and tend to and carry out the wounded. We had no training in guns or weaponry. The United States strictly adhered to the articles of war; medics were not supposed to be combatants.

Forgive me for tooting my own bugle, but I was a good soldier. I was motivated and worked hard at the physical and medical training. You are currently reading the memoir of a former "Soldier of the Month."

My initial training took place at Camp Grant in Rockford, Illinois. Having summoned all my patriotism and courage to enlist and then having trained hard, I expected to be shipped overseas. There, although a medic, I'd be in the midst of combat—doing my best to beat the Nazis and to stay alive. Already, some of the guys in my unit were getting shipped out. But once again the Army had different plans for me. I was enlisted into the ASTP.

The ASTP, the Army Specialized Training Program, was launched early in 1943 "to provide the continuous and accelerated flow of high-grade technicians and specialists needed by the Army." Not every program designed by the military made sense, but this one did. Uncertain how long the war would go on, the

U.S. wanted to ensure that there would be skilled individuals to fill inevitable vacancies in certain fields like engineering, the foreign languages, and medicine.

If you were an enlisted man who had completed basic training, you were eligible to be plucked out from your unit and sent to school. You would remain on active duty and in uniform and you would be expected to continue your service once you had finished your education. With my pre-med background, I was an obvious candidate to bypass the battlefields and, instead, go to medical school. My background, however, did not assure me of ASTP admission. First, I had to pass muster in an interview with a colonel. During our three months of training, we privates had never seen an officer of that rank. On the day before his arrival, we were drilled on how to approach him. Salute, then, "Private Young reporting as instructed."

I passed… with mixed emotions. This switch in plans from combat back to the classroom was anticlimactic. Then again, there were worse places to be stationed than Northwestern University's School of Medicine in my hometown.

Before the academic year began, the Army sent me to Cornell University in Ithaca, New York, to complete my pre-med studies. I studied biological sciences for a semester. As a soldier/student, I lived in a barracks and marched to school.

After Cornell and before classes began at Northwestern, I returned to Rockford. The Army wanted to get all it could from me before I became a doctor. My new assignment? Supervising captive Germans in the prisoner-of-war camp within Camp Grant.

Along with a sergeant, I was in charge of eight Nazi soldiers captured in the North African theatre. Seasoned in battle and self-confident, they were now tasked with cleaning the buildings and grounds of their enemy. But they didn't think they'd be doing that forever. They believed in Aryan superiority and were certain that their countrymen would eventually be victorious and that they would be the first German emissaries in the U.S. (Thanks to my modest understanding of Yiddish, I could understand them and be understood. I don't think they knew I was Jewish—I had no motivation to tell them what the hell I was—and, to be fair, I never heard them spout anti-Semitic ideology). We were enemies, but we weren't angry at each other. Except once.

Among the POWs' duties was spraying to prevent (or combat) rodent and vermin infestations. These prisoner and soldier barracks were prime targets. One day the Germans—apparently wanting to test our will and demonstrate their loyalty to Der Fuhrer—refused to get off the truck. "We will not spray the neger area," said their leader. ("Neger" is the German word for Negro. They weren't using it as a slur.)

The German prisoners thought they had us. If you think about it, many Americans would have fallen for that trap. Remember, in 1943, the service was still, for all practical purposes, segregated and African American soldiers were treated as second-class citizens. Their quarters were isolated from the rest of the camp and considerably more run down.

In addition to thinking we might be in lock step with them ideologically, the Germans also reasoned that we had little leverage. Prisoners of war who refused an order were not going to be shot. Rather, they'd be confined to the camp and lose all the benefits of being on parole, so to speak. Those benefits included a certain amount of freedom to move around their confined area and $1 a day, which they could save in order to buy stuff at the PX—books, candy, and the like.

My sergeant asked me what was going on. He was an older guy, late thirties from rural Minnesota, unenthusiastic about the war, in fact an isolationist of sorts. His goal on these details was to get the work done fast, so we would have two or three hours to relax and do as we pleased in our little field office. He and I got along fine, but weren't the closest of friends.

Cussing was *de rigeur* in the service. But the sarge was a religious man and I had never heard him utter a profanity. When I told him what the Germans were up to, that they felt superior to the blacks and wouldn't get off the truck, he changed character. "Tell those motherfuckers if they don't do that immediately, I'll take them back to camp and they'll never get out," he barked.

I liked that. I hadn't expected him to tolerate the Germans' clear-cut violation of their duties, but I also hadn't expected him to turn angry and profane. This was a lesson for me in making judgments about others.

The Germans didn't understand exactly what he said, but they could read his body language. There was a pause of perhaps thirty seconds and then their leader spouted out an order. The POWs jumped off the truck and sprayed the area.

Not too long after this, I was off to Chicago and medical school. I hadn't seen combat, but I could honestly say I'd fought the Nazis (once) and won.

More than Northwestern awaited me. Jessie Polacheck and I had dated for the past few years. It was an on-again off-again relationship, mostly on. And when I had left for the service there was an unspoken understanding that some time in the future we'd get engaged and marry. I was still only twenty years old. Was the future now?

Three

If you aren't careful, a lot can happen when you are in medical school. I entered Northwestern University in July of 1944 as a newly married private in the United States Army. I received my degree in 1948 as a civilian with two children, Nancy and Polly.

I had no say in ending World War II, and I'm not so sure how much say I had on the domestic front either. Marrying Jessie had been inevitable when I entered the service. The future for those going off to war was uncertain, so many couples tied the knot sooner rather than later. We married in a small, non-religious ceremony in her apartment in 1945. I wore my uniform.

When I started Northwestern, I still wore the uniform. The unmarried military men in our class lived in university housing that the Army and Navy had taken over from NU, primarily Abbott Hall, at Lake Shore Drive and Superior. Because I was married, I lived down the street in a modest one-bedroom apartment at 160 East Superior.

My first term at Northwestern could very well have been my last. After three weeks of classes, a dean called me to his office and told me I was failing.

It wasn't difficult to make a diagnosis. I'd cherished my education at the University of Chicago, but in one important way it hadn't prepared me for NU. Under the system instituted by Robert Hutchins, we had taken one examination at the end of the year for all the marbles. Yes, there were tests and quizzes along the way, but they did not count for anything. Med school was different. We were tested regularly from day one, and the results did count.

The vast majority of my classmates studied for these tests. Still in a U. of C. mindset, I didn't. The dean said that if I didn't start passing these exams, I would be "retired" from the program. That got my attention.

A little history. The first medical school in America predated the Revolutionary War. In 1765, one John Morgan founded this institution at the College of Philadelphia (now the University of Pennsylvania) with a faculty trained at the University of Edinburgh. The school offered lectures and practical experience at the nearby Pennsylvania Hospital founded by Ben Franklin.

Northwestern's School of Medicine cites 1859 as its year of origin, although it did not formally affiliate with the university until 1870. Also in 1870, the Woman's Hospital Medical College opened its doors in Chicago following an unsuccessful effort to integrate three women with the NU men (who objected to the admission of females). Twenty-two years later, it finally affiliated with the university, becoming Northwestern University Woman's Medical School. It closed in 1902, but it wasn't until 1926 that women were admitted to the NU Med School.

There were about 140 people in my medical school class. Almost all of us were in uniform, and almost all of us were male. If not for a scholarship program created by department store magnate Montgomery Ward, there might not have been any women at all. As it was there were only ten. What a far cry from today's medical schools, where some 40 percent of the students are women. (In case you are wondering, World War II was well under way before the U.S. allowed women doctors to be commissioned in the military. Prior to that, the American Medical Association and the surgeons general of the Army and Navy had resisted changes to an existing law that allowed women to serve in the reserves as nurses, but not physicians. When the change finally did materialize in 1943—thanks in large part to a lobbying effort by the American Women's Medical Association—it wasn't because the powers that be were suddenly enlightened. Rather, it was because of the severe shortage of doctors occasioned by the war.)

People of color didn't fare well at NU in the 1940s either. Daniel Hale Williams became the med school's first African American graduate in 1883. He would go on to found Provident Hospital, Chicago's first interracial hospital. (Stay tuned. Provident figures prominently later in my story.) But there weren't any blacks—men or women—in my class.

With no end to the war in sight, those of us who were tapped for the military's specialized training program in late 1943 fully expected to be working for Uncle Sam after we received our MDs. As so many doctors were needed for the war effort, the program was designed to take three years instead of four (although we weren't awarded our MD degrees until we served a one-year internship). We took classes seven days a week instead of five. Sundays were not for rest, but for marching and other military activities.

As I recall our classes were not geared toward the military. Our professors gave us a standard medical school education. At the same time there was no escaping the thought that if you were learning about fractures in an orthopedics class, you might one day be treating fellow soldiers with shattered arms or legs.

I wish I could say that I had a number of memorable professors, but they either weren't that memorable or I simply can't remember. One notable teacher was Loyal Davis. You may know him as the adoptive father of first lady Nancy Reagan.

Dr. Davis, who taught surgery, stood out for several reasons. First and foremost, he was a specialist during a time when there were few specialists. He wasn't merely a general surgeon like other profs, he was a neurosurgeon, one of only a few score in the U.S. at the time. Second, he was the only professor who memorized the names of every student in our class—no small feat. And finally, he worked us hard. He made all of us freshman come in for two hours on Saturday mornings to deal with all kinds of medical questions.

He was not the kind of professor with whom you'd want to have a beer, nor would he have wanted to have one with you. He was conservative, opinionated, distant—not a model I'd emulate. But he was a good teacher.

I have more detailed memories of fellow students, as we were, figuratively anyway, together in the trenches every day. Taking the same courses, taking the same exams, studying together, and marching together tends to create solidarity—just as the military would like. So does sitting in alphabetical order in each class. I came to know the W, X, Y, and Zs quite well.

Although we bonded as soldiers and students, we were of different minds politically. Doctors as a group tend to be conservative; why rock the boat when you are sitting at the captain's table? Many doctors are also the sons or daughters of those conservative doctors. This is something I observe today, and it was even more prevalent in my medical school class. A lot of my fellow students were planning to enter the "family business." Bottom line, the undergrads at the University of Chicago were considerably more liberal than the Northwestern University Medical School Class of 1948, and I was no exception.

You may be wondering if I think men and women who are liberal politically make better doctors than those of the conservative persuasion. Absolutely not. During the training period, particularly the internship and residency, the doctors in training regard their colleagues according to the skills they have acquired. Their motivation coincided very much with the patient's interest. Their esteem resided in how well their patients did.

Our class valedictorian, Rolf Gunnar, and salutatorian, Tom Sheridan, shared little in common, but both became excellent doctors. Rolf was a physician's son, who'd grown up in an affluent suburb west of Chicago. He was quite conservative—a Herbert Hoover Republican—and was on the typical career path, destined to join his father in practice. We were ideological opposites and clashed from time to time, but we were friends and I had great respect for him. He went on to have a brilliant career as chief of cardiology at the University of Illinois, head of the American College of Physicians, and chair of medicine at Cook County. He was ousted from this latter post for ridiculous reasons, and I was approached to succeed him. More on this later.

An only child, Tom was raised by religious Catholic maiden aunts in downstate Illinois. He was one of a handful of classmates not in the military. Because he had an allergy, he was turned down by the Navy.

Tom went through med school without any of the perks that most of us had. We joined "fraternities"—our name for study

24

groups that had copies of old exams. He went through med school working at his father's pharmacy in suburban Skokie. Still he finished number two in our class. He, too, led a distinguished career, becoming chairman of surgery at Michael Reese Hospital. Our lives interlocked dramatically as the years went by, but that is for another chapter, too.

World War II ended during my second year at Northwestern. Germany had surrendered a couple of months before classes began. On August 6, 1945, just a few weeks into the term, the U.S. dropped the first of two atom bombs on Japan. (In the ensuing years I opposed the great enhancement of military destruction, and worked hard for control of the weapon.)

A few weeks later the war was over, but not medical school. I was discharged in 1947 and finished my education thanks to the GI Bill. I sometimes think those who complain about the role of government in our lives forget the impact of this legislation. Before WWII, 5 percent of Americans had college degrees. After the GI Bill was used by returning veterans in the late '40s and early '50s, the U.S. college degree ranks rose to 20 percent and played a great role in America's international hegemony. There is no example of private generosity effecting any similar enhancement of national education.

In my day, as is the case now, state law required would-be doctors to do a one-year internship following medical school. Residencies follow internships. This post-school period is not only the time to improve your skills with more patient contact; it's the time to decide what you want to be when you grow up. Nowadays, just as with about everything else in our society, to the specialists go the spoils. When is the last time you heard someone referred to as a GP (general practitioner) or even as a surgeon (as opposed to an orthopedic surgeon or a cardiac surgeon)? Today, specializing offers the opportunity for bigger bucks. As a result we have far fewer primary care doctors than are needed.

Specialism, as I will explain in detail in the next chapter, was beginning to come into vogue as I finished medical school. But since we were really devoting ourselves to making sure we got through, we, or at least I, gave little thought to it. (Spoiler alert:

When it came time to decide, I didn't have any trouble. I did not want to be a surgeon, nor specialize in a medical area such as dermatology or psychiatry. I wanted to be a general internist, which is a kissing cousin to a general practitioner, except for the fact that you only see adults.)

Of the several Chicago-area hospitals that offered internships, one topped my wish list. Cook County Hospital offered one of the largest and most diversified public training programs in the country. I had clerked there during my third year, doing a couple of one-month-long rotations. It was a mystical place, and I had been enchanted. Along with Bellevue in New York and Los Angeles County, it was one of the three biggest hospitals in the country, with 3,400 beds. (There was always a silly competition to see who had the most beds.) If, like me, you had some notion that you wanted to serve a mass of the masses, this was the place.

County was heaven for anyone wanting to see every affliction, condition, and disease under the sun. It was and remains to this day one of the few institutions where a young doctor can be exposed to every specialty rotation imaginable—from Ob/Gyn to psychiatry to emergency medicine, and a whole array of surgical specialties. My god, there were 100,000 admissions annually, and over 20,000 babies were delivered there every year.

With so much to offer, County always attracted far more applicants than it could accommodate. The hospital took advantage of the law of supply and demand by requiring that interns work for two years before their residency instead of one. This didn't deter me and about 400 other applicants from vying for just 100 spots.

Fortunately, six of those spots were quietly reserved for members of my NU class. When the dean announced this, I jumped, as did five fellow classmates, including Rolf and Tom. We were accepted and began in the summer of 1947.

For the next five years—with the exception of a medical stint in West Virginia in 1951—Cook County Hospital was my home away from home—or maybe it's more accurate to say that my apartment in Hyde Park was my home away from home. I slept in the hospital more nights than I care to remember, leaving Jessie to do the brunt of the child rearing. And there were several children to rear—Nancy, born in 1945; Polly, born in 1947; and Ethan, born in 1952.

Designed in the Beaux-Arts style by architect Paul Gerhardt and completed in 1914, the nine-story, two-block-long County Hospital was located at 1835 W. Harrison Street, about two miles west of Chicago's Loop. To offer you some historical background on this paradise that I entered, allow me to quote extensively from *The Encyclopedia of Chicago*.

"Northwest Territory law and the Illinois General Assembly assigned the care of paupers to the counties. From 1832 until 1866, Cook County fulfilled this obligation by providing a minimum of food and medicine for patients in temporary hospitals or private homes. Physicians and students from Rush Medical School provided free medical care.

A permanent hospital was built by the city of Chicago in 1857. Rush Medical School used the building at 18th and Arnold Streets as a teaching hospital until the Civil War, when it became an army hospital. After the war, the city traded it to Cook County for 160 acres of property which had been used as a reform school. The "Old County Hospital" opened in 1866 in the same building, a three-story brick and limestone structure with "all the modern conveniences," including a knife, saw, and chisel for autopsies.

From its beginning, the Cook County Hospital was a center for medical education. The first internship in the country was started there in 1866. Neither the interns, chosen by competitive examination, nor the attending physicians were paid, but they gained wide experience with every sort of disease.

Corrupt political appointees controlled hospital purchasing and personnel. The physical plant deteriorated and the building became infested with rats and roaches. As city population increased in the 1870s, the hospital became more crowded. Despite public indifference, physicians prevailed upon the county in 1876 to build a new 300-bed facility between Harrison, Polk, Lincoln, and Wood Streets. Political corruption worsened, and, after almost the entire medical staff resigned, the politicians appointed poorly qualified physicians. In 1886 newspaper articles described the patronage-ridden hospital as a "roadhouse" for politicians.

During the early 1900s, political corruption declined, and new civil service laws required that attending physicians pass an examination for staff appointment. As a result, the best surgeons and physicians in Chicago volunteered their services to care for the sick poor and to teach interns. A huge new hospital opened in 1914, anchoring a complex that eventually grew to (over) 3,000 beds.

From the 1920s until immediately after World War II, the Cook County Hospital, despite continued political problems and a seriously deteriorating physical plant, was regarded as one of the world's great teaching hospitals. Interns, residents, and graduate physicians came for experience and to see outstanding medical and surgical work. Scientific innovations included the world's first blood bank and the surgical fixation of fractures."

Interns, residents, and graduate physicians. Interns were those of us who had just finished medical school. We were counseled by residents (who had completed their internships). Still higher on the food chain were the attendings—respected physicians who with very few exceptions were on the faculties at various medical schools in the Chicago area. Attendings wore street garb, suits or dresses, while the rest of us wore white jackets.

While we interns rotated from ward to ward, the residents and attendings remained in the ward of their chosen field. These included the pediatric hospital, surgical, medical wards, and specialty wards (for example, the admitting ward, which was really an intensive care unit, until patients were stabilized enough to be sent to their ward). By the end of our two years, we had spent about twelve months in the surgical field and twelve months in the clinical field.

Interns were also assigned supplementary duty in the Emergency Room every three or four weeks. Whatever your rotation responsibilities—caring for thirty sick people or doing surgery—you were expected to put that to the side temporarily and handle emergencies. It was like KP (kitchen police) duty in the Army, except our turf was the ER, not the mess hall.

An Emergency Room story: In the ER, we worked fast. We got to what the problem was and distributed the patient to a clinic or admitted him/her if it was serious enough. We had several alternatives. One day, I sent a patient from the ER up to Ear, Nose, and Throat (ENT). A few minutes later a doctor from ENT called and asked me to come up right away. When I arrived, the doctor said, "This guy says he's your patient."

"I remember him," I said. "I sent him here."

"Yeah you sent him here. Let the patient tell you what's wrong."

The patient said with all seriousness, "My nose is getting longer and longer."

I looked at the doctor, smiled, and said, "That's ENT."

County had the first trauma unit in the country. This was a space devoted to people who were injured by gunshots or automobile crashes or by jumping through windows, or by almost any other accidental or self-inflicted injury you can imagine. Trauma doesn't have to wait years or decades to mature like a disease. It's right then and there. There was no pause in nearly anything at County, least of all trauma. Men, women, and children flowed into and through the unit night and day.

**

County was divided into departments (such as Medicine, Pediatrics, and Surgery), each of which had a chairperson, almost exclusively male in those days. Chairs had quite a bit of autonomy… as long as they didn't ruffle the feathers of the fellow who ruled the roost, the legendary Dr. Karl A. Meyer.

Meyer, a skilled surgeon, was the administrator of the hospital, appointed by the elected County Commissioners, card-carrying members of the Democratic Party Machine. He held that title for fifty-three years. That is not a typo. From 1914 to 1967, Cook County Hospital was Karl Meyer's fiefdom. During his tenure County became one of the most highly regarded training hospitals in the country… and one of the most political.

You can't be a political appointee—even if you are in a profession like medicine—without being a politician yourself. And Meyer, a short, nondescript ruler who seldom smiled, was a master practitioner.

Holding power over the attendings—who had wards of their own—as well as department chairs, Meyer had a subservient following within the hospital. Being an attending physician was a big deal—for the medical school with which the doctor was affiliated and, of course, the doctor himself or herself. The post was a steppingstone to a medical school professorship and distinction in the Chicago medical world.

Attendings gained their appointments by taking an exam. But once in place, they realized that antagonizing the powers that be was not in their self-interest. This did not make them evil people; it simply made them "company men" or women. And while some may have been more interested in having the title than serving the patients, many were dedicated and willing to spend long hours at the hospital teaching interns and residents.

Meyer held as much sway with the County Board and the Machine as he did with the doctors. County was a major employer of patronage workers and an ongoing plum for politically connected vendors and construction companies. Over the years, Meyer expanded his turf, becoming, for a while, president of the University of Illinois Board of Trustees.

While today County's population is overwhelmingly African American and Latino, many patients in the 1940s were immigrants from Eastern Europe, particularly Poland. During Meyer's tenure, the hospital admirably administered to the poor. Less well known is the fact that the hospital also administered to the not so poor, most of whom had political connections. Because the doctors were first rate, local pols often sent their own family members and friends and patronage workers to County for surgery or other treatment. These special patients had their own special ward, and the higher-ups in the hospital administration followed their progress closely.

"Now a lot of people come here with slips from their precinct captain or their ward committeeman or even their congressman," the hospital's medical director told our incoming class of interns. "Those slips say the bearer is a worthy citizen and you should admit them to the hospital. Now you and I know they don't need those slips. But they think they do. So there's no sense tearing up those slips or criticizing the precinct captain. Just tell the patient you will take good care of them."

Thus were we oriented to the critical role County Hospital played as a service expression for the political Machine. Those who believed such a note was needed further believed they owed a political debt to their benefactor. So the medical director was giving our new team an instruction, reinforced through residency: the Organization's interest was to assure that its minions assumed the hospital's services were a benefit or reward for political fidelity.

Patients who required no hospital care (often unwanted elderly relatives) were regularly admitted after a visit or phone call to the warden's office. "Admit, per Warden," was an override familiar to the Emergency Room doctors. No one ever challenged this abuse of terribly over-strained resources. Physicians-in-training, who would fight for their sick patients as a tigress for her cubs, were fully compliant, learning early on to "render unto Caesar," even if Caesar subverted the hospital's mission.

The VIP ward was located on the sixth floor of the pediatric hospital. The remainder of the wards were spread out all over. There were two sides to a ward: male and female (with the obvious exception of the Ob/Gyn ward). In the late 1940s, as I recall, a ward ordinarily had forty beds. When business got good, however, the number jumped to sixty. And when business got really good, there were 100 beds.

There was no such thing as a private room. Each ward had a space of six to eight beds for the most seriously ill people, which is a euphemism for people who are going to die. But by and large County featured large, open wards.

It was too cold in the winter, too hot in the summer. There were no private bathrooms. Patients used bedpans or, if ambulatory, walked to the part of the ward where there were toilets. It was pretty gruesome.

As interns, our rotations lasted up to six months. On my first day, I was assigned to Ob/Gyn. Within 30 minutes I had assisted in the delivery of my first baby. I was put in a room with women in labor and told to get to work. This was after all "Normal" OB (as opposed to "Pathological" OB—a different assignment during the rotation).

What if I had a question? Or needed help? There may have been a resident in the room for the first few deliveries, on call just to make sure I didn't botch things up. But after that I was on my own, though during this rotation and the ones that followed, I learned that I could call on the residents for backup. Medically, not administratively, they ran the show. Some had been at County for five years and knew as much as anyone is going to know in their specialty.

Of course when you are doing something for the first time or encountering a situation that you didn't read about in your medical school books, you try not to let your patient know you are lost. Did these patients suffer because we were totally green? Because with little or no supervision (or sleep) we were trying to handle thirty sick people? At first, perhaps, but we had other backup besides the residents.

The nurses had been there for years, seen just about everything, and were extremely helpful—especially if you treated them with the respect they deserved. They'd seen a million Quentin Youngs come there without a penny's worth of skill. So in Ob/Gyn the nurses protected the mothers, and in the other wards the nurses protected their particular patients.

My Ob/Gyn rotation was divided into three twenty-day assignments. During one of those terms we saw "normal" patients. During another term, we saw "pathological" patients—those pregnant women who were sick with heart disease, hypertension, or kidney disease. Finally, and most interesting, we had a "septic" OB stint. Septic here meant women suffering the effects of incomplete abortions that were criminally performed or self-induced.

The sequence of those twenty-day terms was arbitrary. You didn't necessarily start with the normal and work your way to the most difficult. You were assigned to whatever spot needed to be filled. Luck of the draw, my first service was with women who were judged normal on admission.

We worked 24 hours on and then 24 hours off, then rinsed and repeated. There was never a shortage of mothers. I averaged about fifteen deliveries a day and sometimes brought as many as twenty newborns into the world on a 24-hour shift.

Every once in a while there was a rare spell when nobody was in labor. But by and large you worked 24 hours, staggered to bed, slept, sort of recovered and then went back for another day. County featured long corridors of bedrooms for its doctors. Many interns lived there around the clock, but I went home to my family about every other day.

In recent years, interns and others lobbied for changes in their working conditions. Sixty-five years ago there was no such move-ment. I suppose the residents could have initiated something, but they were able to sleep more than the interns; if you needed them, you woke them up. Moreover, since they'd gone through it and survived, darned if they were going to give us a pass. A 24-hour shift was a kind of crazy initiation into a way of life that had ex-isted for decades.

The intern/residency was in many ways a morbid plight—a plight for which we received room and board but no pay our first year and about $100 per month our second year. In my class of 100, we had a suicide, a natural death, and several serious illness-es, including tuberculosis and polio. Then, as today, the hospital is not the best place to be if you want to stay healthy.

Medical school did not offer a class in bedside manners. So how do you learn them? I can only speak for myself, and since the eye cannot behold itself, I may be an unreliable narrator.

First off, I had been "political" since age thirteen. This was a period of a variety of "lefty" causes—notably attempts to address fascism abroad and the overt racial discrimination that blacks ex-perienced: slavery in the early years, racial discrimination since the Civil War. So I came to County aware that poor people were generally denied dignity and respect.

I tried to let that worldview inform my interaction with each patient. But I don't want to exaggerate. I can't say that when I was seeing my ninth patient in an hour that I was the most pleasant person in the world. Still, I don't think I was too bad. (And here's a secret: if you treat patients in a respectful way and indicate a sincere interest in what's wrong with them, you'll get a better history than if you quickly override any conversation.)

I was also able to learn a lot about dealing with patients by watching and talking with my peers and superiors. We interns spoke with each other about everything. And when we rotated through the Department of Medicine and some other departments like Ob/Gyn, Pediatrics, and Surgery, we followed residents, staff physicians, and attendings on their grand rounds each week. Here, we not only learned about medical conditions from experts, we'd see how the more experienced doctors dealt with patients—sometimes for better, sometimes for worse.

In the same way that we young doctors developed our bedside manners based on our own worldviews and by observing others, we learned how to deal with death. At a place like County where there was such a high volume of patients, many seriously ill or terminal, the patients and their families tended to look at us doctors—even the lowliest of us—as almost god-like. Their lives were in your hands and they wanted to believe that we had a kind of supernatural power. Subtly and sometimes unconsciously a doctor learns how to use that impression.

Example: You often know when you see a new patient that he or she has a fatal disease and very few days to live. In all likelihood, the patient is not the proper person to talk to; you have to tell the family, parents, husband, wife, whomever. And so, you slowly develop a technique and skill in letting people know what the news is. Part of that is not to tell too much at one time. People can't process this, particularly if it is a new development. If the patient suddenly became ill, you can't tell them, "Well, Papa's gonna die in two days." Instead, you do your best to describe the process and explain what you are going to do and what they can do.

It's an odd image, but I thought of this as similar to slicing salami. You don't want to swallow the salami in one bite. Remarkably—and this is not a matter of sophistication or education—the family will ask as much as they can take at the time. Maybe the next day they'll ask you more. What I'm saying is that part of the skill of communication is learning how to respond to the family's unanswered questions. That's part of doctoring that doesn't get enough attention.

It's also important to address how a doctor responds when a patient dies. Obviously the reaction varies with the circumstance. It's one thing to have a ninety-year-old guy who has been sick for the preceding ten years die and quite another to lose a young person who has what seemed a treatable disease where the diagnosis either wasn't made in time or at all.

Each scenario presented itself many times at County. Blunders happen at any institution and maybe even more so at public hospitals where so much responsibility is given so quickly to freshly trained younger people. You can never be happy with that, yet over time you somehow build up your defenses. You can't mourn every patient who dies on your watch. If you did, you'd be paralyzed, unable to have the confidence necessary to treat someone.

Any doctor, particularly one working at a place like County, knows patient death is inevitable. *When* it happens is another issue; maybe you can intervene. If it becomes clear that things you didn't do or did do contributed to a patient's failure, you are self-aware, even self-critical. But I don't want to exaggerate that. I don't think County residents who had plenty of experience with deadly events cried most of the time. I think survival demanded that they have a defense against self-doubt.

So at what stage do young doctors begin to realize they aren't god-like or possessed of supernatural powers? To tell the truth, I'm not sure we ever forego it... at least not entirely. I think most physicians, maybe all to some degree, see themselves as the intermediary in people's health or illness—for the patient himself or herself or the family. Part of our mystique is that for hundreds if not thousands of years, doctors and the keepers of religion were the same person. It was only in modern times that authority shifted from the religious to the medical and these callings got separated into healers and faith-givers.

Whether true or not, County's patients thought they were being treated by the best doctors in the world. By and large, they did not have the feeling that they were being abused or mistreated. County would be a perfect setting for that to develop, but it didn't.

I tell the story about a conversation I had when I was chair of the Department of Medicine more than twenty years after my internship. One day I was in the critical care ward getting to know a new patient. I looked over his chart. He was a real old guy, suffering from heart failure, which required he sit up to breathe, and I engaged him with conversation as best I could.

"I'm Dr. Young. So tell me why you came here."

"Well I was a sick man, I came here sick."

"Yes," I said, "but your ambulance passed twenty hospitals on your way here. Why did you come to County?"

He said, "I always come here."

You can understand why I was asking him. "Yeah, but you came so far. You could have gone to any nearby hospital."

And he said, "This is *my* hospital. I always come here."

And that's very telling. Psychologically he thought that this was *his* hospital.

Not to be cynical, but it wasn't his hospital. It was Mayor Daley's and County board President George Dunne's hospital and a very important cog in the political machine.

The man didn't think that public housing was his or the grade school where his kid or grandchild went was his. But he did think this hospital was his hospital.

That's a lesson to be remembered.

In 1996, a 7th grader named Emily Hagen interviewed me for a paper she was writing about the history of Cook County Hospital. Did County inspire me? she wondered. The hospital, I responded, "was like a loving mother with arms outstretched to embrace all who sought her care. Without barrier and with no exclusionary questions asked, County stood poised to help all comers and usually the care was very good."

And what did I learn at County? "I am convinced that until we, as a nation, have a system of universal health care, including everyone—everybody in, nobody out—until we provide that, we as a society must provide care through a system like County."

Sadly, all these years later, this is still the case.

Four

Having read this far you may be wondering: where's that Quentin Young, the agitator? Where's the troublemaker that so worried the FBI, House Un-American Activities Committee, and others? Well, you have come to the right chapter.

During the three years of my residency and the beginning years of my practice, I joined with some fine men and women to lobby for national health insurance and to try and do something about the racial discrimination that existed in medical school admissions policies, staff privileges and patient admissions at Chicago hospitals, and within the AMA itself. But before chronicling those efforts, allow me a few words about my residency—and one word in particular: specialization.

As noted earlier, specialization was just coming into vogue when I started medical school. The return of young doctors from World War II sparked the trend. In the military these guys (and a few gals) had seen that rank had its privileges and specialty had its rank. So the old notion of doing a one-year internship and then hanging out your shingle as a GP was beginning to decline.

The demise was hastened by post-war federal policy, namely the subsidizing of full-time faculty in the med schools. This virtually guaranteed the growth of specialism because the medical students' new peer models were specialists—who, because they chose to go academic, were making a statement that placed research and education above practice.

This was a terribly important cultural and academic phenomenon. Who picks the incoming students? The faculty. Who trains the students and tells them what to do with their careers as they're leaving? The faculty, or, more precisely, the faculty specialists.

Was the death of the general practice model mourned? By some, perhaps. But it was a quiet passing, one that sort of crept up on us. I don't think there was an awareness that anything was happening. Neither at Northwestern nor County were we subjected to pep talks or even scientific talks with the message, "We must end this primitive, useless form of generalist care."

A transformation was taking place, but the participants weren't hyperaware of it. We didn't grasp that we were part of a profound shift in health care arrangements that reflected at once the explosion of technology, the expansion of health insurance, and other events.

As a medical student, trainee, and, later, as junior faculty, I really didn't have a sense—as I have had with other issues in health care—that change was a comin' and that we should resist it or facilitate it. I did, however, know what I wanted to do.

When doing internal medicine as an intern at County, I'd relished being the first physician to see the patient and the challenge of figuring out what the hell was going on. *Fix it yourself and be good or, at the appropriate time, refer out to a specialist.* That was the life of an internist, and I liked that. The internist infantry was the queen of battle. We had the task of seeing the patients, taking the stories they told, examining them, and trying to make a good plan to make them well.

(Internal medicine, by the way, was and still is a specialty, albeit the one that came the closest to the generalist model. It offered Board certification and took three more years of training after internship.)

It's fair to ask if during this period my fellow doctors and I looked down upon the generalist, the historic doc, the GP. That's tricky. The teaching centers had an acronym for such practitioners, LMD—Local Medical Doctor—and it was not spoken with reverence. LMDs were considered mediocre. Such judgment was not rendered because they were unspecialized, but because we thought they didn't know as much as we did. Four extra years of training and doctoring at a public hospital can teach you a lot.

This I can say with certainty about my residency: I slept better and saw more of my family than I had as an intern. I also had more responsibility and was more firmly located on my career path. Everything I did was related to internal medicine, as opposed to surgery or other specialties. I either worked on a ward with patients who had already been admitted, or in a clinic with outpatients, or provided consultation. When other parts of the hospital needed a medical opinion, a resident like me would come and give it and then transfer a patient or order tests or procedures. We also decided whether or not to admit patients whom we saw in the clinics. County filled its beds with people who came to the ER or those clinics.

Our authority grew year by year. Much of the first year of residency was spent in "basic science," aka working in the pathology department. Here, I caught a break. I was approached by the incumbent researcher who was studying urinary potassium excretion in patients with advanced hypertensive cardiovascular disease. Would I like to help him instead of doing the traditional first year of residency training?

This seemed like a more interesting alternative, so I accepted. The supervisor of the research, Dr. William Hoffman, County's director of clinical laboratories, then suggested I approach the University of Illinois Chicago campus graduate school to see if this work could lead to a masters in science degree. Great idea!

I remember the interview with the chief of graduate research at U. of I. vividly. He asked what courses I intended to take. I said, "None." He was dismayed and he made some suggestions. I said, "I already took those classes." He asked where. I said. "Northwestern Medical School."

"You've been to med school?"

"Yes."

"Well, in that case, Doctor, we'd be glad if you simply attended the Wednesday noon conference whenever you could."

Even greater idea! I did attend some of those Wednesday seminars.

By the end of my residency, the study on potassium was published and actually won the state medical society prize, $500, for graduate research. Based on publication—not attendance—I was awarded the masters of science.

In addition to becoming an expert on potassium excretions, I learned quite a bit about pulmonary medicine during my residency. I spent a portion of my time at Oak Forest Hospital in the south suburbs. Once called the "Cook County Poor Farm," Oak Forest specialized in long-term care. In the late 1940s and early 1950s, that translated to tuberculosis care. Indeed, of the 12,000 beds in the Chicago area at that time, some 4,000 were dedicated to TB, which required isolation from the general population until the introduction of a drug called isoniazid, INH for short.

Three of us at a time were on service at Oak Forest Hospital. We each had 100 patients, some of whom were recovering and some of whom were dying. I still remember one particular bed where it seemed like there was a new patient every day. "How many people have you seen die in that bed?" I asked the patient who shared the room.

"About 100 head," he said. As if they were cattle.

During the second year of my residency—1951—I had the opportunity to leave Chicago for a more exotic locale. I thought I was going to Southeast Asia. Instead, I ended up in West Virginia.

What happened? Originally, I volunteered and was assigned to be part of a sixty-person professional medical team, recruited into the public health service, slated to travel to a variety of sites in the Orient, including Burma (now called Myanmar), Dutch East Indies, and Formosa (now called Taiwan). Sponsored by the U.S. State Department, our purpose was to engage the public health issues in the region and thereby win over the countries from "anti-American" regimes.

Before leaving we spent three months in Boston learning about those health issues at Harvard's School of Public Health. Toward the end of the training period, about fifteen of us were told that we could not attend classes until "clearance" was obtained from the State Department. In the days that followed, most were "cleared." Not me.

All sixty of us went to Washington, D.C. for "political orientation." There the head of the U.S. Public Health Service told six of us that we had been declared "unacceptable for the mission." Genuinely apologetic that we had trained for three months only to be blackballed, he assured us that the State Department, not the Health Service, had made that decision.

He asked each of us if we knew of any reason for such actions. I told him that I'd been disagreeing with State Department policy for years. I did not like the fact that these Southeast Asian countries were dominated by European masters. Post WWII, the independence movement had grown throughout the region, and I supported it.

Although denied an adventure in Southeast Asia, we were given other options. The Health Service could place us within the U.S. borders (where presumably we could do no harm!) in a public health hospital, in the federal Indian Health Service, or in venereal disease control. I chose the last because effective medication for gonorrhea and syphilis was just coming into use.

Following intensive training in Hot Springs, Arkansas, I was assigned to work in West Virginia. I lived in South Charleston, at the site of an old National Youth Act post, long since closed. Jessie, her mother, and our children joined me.

Each week I traveled around the state by car, starting at public health sites in the north, then moving south. I would identify those with the diseases and arrange for their transfer to South Charleston for treatment. Usually I drove them myself.

It's worth noting that our main targets, syphilis and gonorrhea, could now, in 1952, be cured by one or two injections of penicillin; but the older regimen with less effective drugs administered over a six-week period was still the order of the day in treatment centers nationwide. The treatment protocol would be modified later and be based on penicillin therapy. This was valuable work, helping me learn how to deal with public health problems.

There was an additional benefit: Thanks to conversations on our jaunt back to South Charleston, I learned a great deal about working people, mostly coal miners. One patient in his seventies described going into the mines as a child with his father. He explained that the miners then didn't have a shift defined by hours, but rather by the amount of coal they were expected to bring out. They often stayed underground well past the typical eight-hour day. And so thanks to my VD patients, my education continued. I gained a more profound understanding of workplace exploitation and exhaustion.

After my public health service, I returned to County to complete my residency. Our responsibilities increased with years of residency training. In my final, fourth year, I became chief resident, meaning that I made consultations and supervised the younger internal medicine trainees.

And now for the agitating. While in medical school and then at County, I was a proud, card-carrying member of the Association of Interns and Medical Students. Formed in 1941, AIMS had the audacity to lobby for national health insurance, the end to racial and gender discrimination in medical schools, and better policies to address unwanted pregnancies, slum-bred tuberculosis, and other health issues. Add to this the fact that we were allied with the labor movement and you have a prescription for being a pain to the medical establishment—even if AIMS wasn't in even half the medical schools in the nation and our membership was relatively small.

Nonetheless, feeling the heat, the AMA national leadership in 1949 instructed all medical school deans to advise students that they wouldn't graduate if they were affiliated with AIMS. Seeing their careers pass before their eyes, many young men and women quit AIMS. By 1952 the organization was finished. At the same time, the AMA created its own more reliably conservative adjunct, the Student American Medical Association. (Some seven years later, SAMA would assert its independence and disassociate itself from the AMA and rename itself the American Medical Students Association, AMSA, an organization which flourishes to this day.)

I don't think it's a coincidence that the AMA's witch-hunt coincided with the McCarthyism of the day. That heinous movement to ferret out anyone who ever had anything to do with the left extended well beyond government and Hollywood to the halls of Cook County Hospital. After Ethel and Julius Rosenberg were convicted in 1951 of passing atomic secrets to the Soviets, a worldwide clemency movement sprang up. Among those joining the effort were a small number of doctors at County, including me. My classmate Tom Sheridan, who was president of the house staff, went to the mailroom and asked that a notice of a "Clemency for the Rosenbergs" meeting be distributed. Hospital head Karl Meyer was furious. He demanded Tom apologize or lose his residency. Tom refused. Fortunately for Tom, in the middle of this, Pope Pius XII announced his support of clemency. As the Machine that employed Meyer had a large Catholic contingency and relationship with the Church, Meyer decided not to test his power against that of the Pope. Tom survived.

Before AIMS disbanded it worked hard to establish a national health insurance plan and to eliminate racial discrimination in medical schools and in post-med school training programs.

"I consider it socialism. It is to my mind the most socialistic measure this Congress has ever had before it."

Sound familiar? No, this was not the rant of a contemporary opponent of Obamacare. Rather, this was Senator Robert Taft, Republican of Ohio, railing against President Harry Truman's national health care initiative in the mid-to-late-1940s.

Despite the support of AIMS and others in the progressive movement, Truman's plan for universal comprehensive health insurance was doomed for several reasons. First, the Republicans took control of Congress in 1946, and they tapped into a postwar, anti-Communist fervor. Anything that could be branded as straight out of the Soviet constitution had little chance of success. One pamphlet read: "Would socialized medicine lead to socialization of other phases of life? Lenin thought so. He declared socialized medicine is the keystone to the arch of the socialist state."

Joining the Republican opposition was the medical establishment, notably the AMA and the American Hospital Association. Doctors will become slaves, cried the AMA, though nothing could have been further from the truth. Under Truman's proposed plan, doctors were allowed to select their method of payment: fee-for-service, group practice, or other models.

In 1948, fearful that the newly elected Truman might use

his victory to push through national health insurance, the AMA tacked $25 on to members' dues for use in a lobbying effort. (In 1945 they had spent $1.5 million on lobbying—at the time the most costly lobbying effort in American history.)

You can guess what happened. Despite attempts at compromise, the Truman forces—and the American people—lost. Private insurance won the day and the next 65 years (with the exception of Medicare).

The effort to eliminate discrimination in the medical profession was more successful, though that battle, too, continues. Along with my friend, an African American surgeon named Clyde Phillips, I was co-chair of AIMS' Regional Committee on Discrimination in Medicine. In 1949, we wrote a letter to the medical directors at eight Chicago hospitals, including Cook County, Michael Reese and Billings (the University of Chicago). It read:

"As an administrator in an outstanding metropolitan hospital, you are in daily contact with the pressing health needs of Chicago's Negro population. Though grounded in poverty and slums, this problem has been heightened by consistent limitations placed on the training of Negro physicians. These restrictions are reflected at the medical school level by approximately 150 Negroes among the 5,000 or more students graduating annually. And in the class of June '49 there were but 14 Negro MDs produced by all the medical schools excepting Howard and Meharry, the two Negro institutions.

Still more obstacles confront the Negro medical aspirants. A recent survey revealed that they must choose from among 158 available internships, and these mostly in small, Negro hospitals. A similar condition obtains in regard to residences. Obviously, physicians trained in the best medical centers can do much to ameliorate the health needs of their people. Your hospital is presently choosing its house-staff for 1950. We urge you give special attention to qualified Negro applicants for intern and resident positions.

We in medicine have an ultimate obligation to the community. By training young Negro physicians, (your hospital) will benefit a long neglected portion of our population. Our Committee is most interested in your action on this vital matter and would certainly welcome an exchange of ideas."

The response of the health industry was that they were unaware of any discrimination.

**

As our residencies ended, my mates and I went off in a variety of directions. Almost all of us went into private practice in Chicago and Illinois, but in other locations also. Most people went back to their hometowns.

My plan was to set up a practice in a neighborhood near the steel mills on Chicago's far South Side and serve blue collar workers. Color me too idealistic. No one would rent me space. In my mind the potential landlords made their decisions for political reasons. They didn't want a doctor on the premises who would be treating union men and women.

And so I ended up on more familiar, welcoming turf—Hyde Park. There I shared office space with another doctor who'd been in practice for about five years, Lou Popuch.

I needed to have an income to support Jessie and our three kids, so while I was building the practice, I took a salaried position as a junior attending physician at Oak Forest Hospital (part of the County system). I spent my mornings there with long-term care TB patients and then hurried back to Hyde Park.

My practice served men and women of all colors, ages, and financial means. Business was pretty good from the beginning. Having lived in the area all my life, I had many friends there, some of whom became my patients. Some steelworkers did come from their neighborhood to me, as well.

It's standard operating procedure for a doctor in private practice to apply to local hospitals for "privileges." If your patients need to be hospitalized, you need to be able to visit them and treat them or consult with those who are treating them. I applied to Provident Hospital, Michael Reese Hospital, and Woodlawn Hospital. And there's an important story to be told about each one.

As noted earlier, Provident had been founded by Daniel Hale

Williams, the first African American to graduate from Northwestern Medical school (1883) and one of the few black physicians of his time in Chicago. Thanks to the book *African Americans in Science*, by Carey and Tucker, I can offer this history: "The doors for the then 12-bed hospital and nurse training facility designed to serve the poor and sick on the South and West side opened in 1891 in a three-story brick house at 29th and Dearborn. Ten years later it had 65 beds, was treating 6,000 patients per year and had moved to 36th and Dearborn. The great Frederick Douglass helped in the fundraising effort. By 1915, black patients made up the vast majority of the hospital's patient population."

Provident moved to the location I knew, 426 East 51st St., in 1933. That's when the University of Chicago sold the hospital a run-down building that had been the site of an ob/gyn hospital Chicago Lying-in. It was moving into new, state-of-the-art quarters on the university campus. This transaction was not unusual for the times, when medical facilities were separate but unequal. In major cities like Chicago, the worn-out white hospital was often given over to the black community.

In 1947, Montague Cobb, an African American anthropologist and MD at Howard University, wrote a wonderful article titled "Old Clothes to Sam: America's Segregated Hospital System." Dr. Cobb—gifted, motivated, and pretty militant—showed that there were eleven U.S. cities that had a "black hospital" like Provident. In each of these cities, the presence of that black hospital virtually guaranteed the segregation of the black physicians; with few exceptions, they did not have privileges at the other hospitals in the cities. In the American cities that had no black hospitals, the integration, such as it was, happened faster.

When I received my privileges in 1952, Provident was still Chicago's black hospital. The place was a mess. Disgusting. Primitive. From another era. As I recall there were only two bathrooms on each floor. Sick people had to crawl to the toilet or use a bedpan. Provident did not enjoy a good reputation among many black patients. They knew that it was a run-down place, and it was rarely their first choice. Most preferred the much larger County Hospital even if it was further away from home.

My education continued: here was what the black physician and patient had to put up with in America circa 1952. I couldn't have learned this without being there on a regular basis.

There may have been a few white doctors who were consultants at Provident, but I don't think there were any besides me on staff. Having made friends with several black physicians through our attempts to end racial discrimination, I didn't get too many, *What the hell are you doing here?* stares. Or: *Why don't you go to your own hospital?*

There were plenty of reasons for black doctors to resent a white doctor who could go elsewhere instead of coming to their hospital. On the other hand, these doctors had been victimized by racial exclusion and didn't want to perpetuate it in reverse. I can't complain about how I was treated at Provident.

While few of the black doctors on the staff at Provident had the opportunity to join the staffs at many other hospitals in Chicago, I did. My first choice was Michael Reese, located at 29th and Ellis, just west of Lake Michigan. Arguably the best hospital in the area, it was also at one time the largest, with 2,400 beds. Courtesy of Hitler, the staff included many top-notch European-born Jewish doctors who had fled or survived the Nazis.

My interview at Reese was not going well and I was on the road to being rejected when I happened to mention that I had a good deal of experience in treating tuberculosis. TB was still a serious problem, and the institution had made a substantial commitment to treating patients with the disease. Reese had a satellite hospital in Winfield, Illinois, offering inpatient treatment to deal with tuberculosis. During this period, few doctors had the experience I had gained while at County.

Suddenly, I was in at Reese—if not through the back door, then through the side door, with an appointment in "chest medicine." As part of the bargain, I had to spend one week a month out in Winfield. It was a helluva drive, taking two hours each way. I also continued to see my private patients in the afternoons in Hyde Park.

There were only five or six doctors in chest medicine at what was then about a 1,000-bed hospital. As a very junior person, I was responsible for doing three or four clinics a week at Reese. As I'll discuss in the next chapter, such duties, as interesting as they were, served to reinforce my conviction that the joy and comfort and satisfaction lay mostly in seeing all kinds of people with all kinds of illnesses.

Woodlawn was the third hospital at which I received staff privileges. It was an old, decrepit hospital, but it had the virtue of being just across the Midway from the University of Chicago medical center. As a result, a few university doctors were on staff, raising the standard to a pretty high level. I applied because the hospital was in my neighborhood.

Woodlawn figures prominently in the story of the battle to integrate Chicago's hospitals. Some more alphabet soup: CEDC-MI was the acronym for the Committee to End Discrimination in Chicago's Medical Institutions. The organization, which I helped found while still at County in 1951, was comprised largely of doctors and nurses and other people in the health professions—black and white—who were deeply concerned about the sanctioned discriminatory practice in health care that was indefensible from any moral or medical viewpoint. Some people were slighted by such a pattern; others lost their lives.

Separate but equal was official hospital policy in Chicago. And to make matters even worse, it was in reality a policy of separate and *dramatically unequal*, impossible to reconcile with the American pretentions of equality and access. Impossible to tolerate at any time, but particularly after African Americans had accepted their own second-class status to fight for America in World War II.

CEDCMI obviously didn't want for examples. At any given time there would be a terrible story: A black person with insurance—and there were many such people, thanks to coverage provided through union membership in auto, steel and meat packing—was sent from a private hospital to County. Worse, somebody perished because he/she wasn't given admission to a particular hospital due to discrimination. In short, there was an ongoing oppression, and we had several people in the field documenting events.

The leader of our movement, CEDCMI's chairman, was the late Dr. Arthur G. Falls. An African American, he was a prominent surgeon and had been chief of staff at Provident Hospital. Arthur had experienced the full brunt of discrimination and refused to suffer the fools still purveying racism. He was a devout Catholic. Believe it or not, when his son was to be confirmed, the church insisted on separating him and other black children from the white children in the ceremony. As committed as he was to his faith, Arthur nonetheless refused to let his son be confirmed.

Arthur was an excellent leader, an articulate man with a wonderful sense of humor and great laugh. He was that rarity, a black graduate of Northwestern Medical School (Class of 1923, the year of my birth). His wife Lillian, a social worker of considerable reputation, was also involved with CEDCMI.

CEDCMI focused its attention on the remarkable pattern of racial exclusion in Chicago's seven medical schools and 68 hospitals. As Arthur noted in a 1963 article titled, "The Search for Negro Medical Students," there were only fourteen black students at these institutions in 1951. Confronted with these numbers, the deans of these schools promised to welcome "qualified minority students." This was a small victory that required constant monitoring, and in his article Arthur lamented that the number had actually dropped from fourteen to ten over the ensuing twelve years.

At the same time we lobbied the med schools, we began approaching the city's hospitals, which were systematically denying admission to patients because of race. As it turned out, the case that turned the tide in our favor did not involve racial discrimination. Still, it shone a light on despicable practices and that light eventually got us to the end of the tunnel.

The case: On January 18, 1954, Laura Lingo, the five-month-old child of European immigrants, was scalded by hot oil from an overturned vaporizer. Her mother Irene rushed her to nearby Woodlawn Hospital. When Mrs. Lingo was unable to pay a $100 cash deposit, the hospital refused to admit the severely injured baby. Laura was sent to Cook County Hospital, where she died the next day.

Did Woodlawn's actions cause the child's death? Obviously the hospital's conduct didn't help, and the doctor who treated Laura at County suggested she should never have been transported. The Cook County Coroner launched an investigation into the death, and the Cook County states attorney said he would examine whether hospitals given tax-free status were providing the level of charitable care required by law. In response, a spokesman for Chicago area hospitals told the press, "Unlimited care of the poor would wreck the hospitals."

The Lingo case captured the attention of the public and of CEDCMI. On February 2, I was one of six people from the organization, five of whom were doctors, to call for action in a letter published by the *Chicago Tribune*. After noting that CEDCMI had been investigating discrimination for three years, we stated that, "We have found a bad situation exists in regard to discriminatory practices against minority groups." We applauded the current investigations, but said, "They should be broadened to include discrimination against patients because of race or color."

Hoping to avoid future Laura Lingo cases, we argued for decentralization of Cook County Hospital, with branches in various sections of the city and/or reimbursement to private hospitals by the city for unpaid emergency hospitalization expenses. New York City already had such a plan.

And then the centerpiece of our effort: "We also recommend public support of legislation at the city and state levels to remedy and prevent other possible tragedies. This could be accomplished by denying licensure and tax exemption to hospitals that turn away patients solely because of their financial situation, race, creed, or color."

We did not mention Woodlawn by name in the letter. We weren't trying to let the hospital off the hook, but our focus was on the system in general. Nevertheless, there was fallout. The hospital revoked my privileges.

Everyone knew discrimination existed—except apparently the Chicago Hospital Council. This umbrella organization said it did not track patients and didn't believe there was systematic discrimination. There was plenty of anecdotal evidence before the Lingo case, but we realized we needed hard evidence to back up our allegations, numbers to demonstrate who was being treated (and not treated) where.

Numbers. Births and deaths in hospitals are recorded on certificates. Such certificates include names, dates, and—how about this?—race. Granted such certificates aren't smoking-gun-proof of a policy to discriminate, but they are hard to argue with; there can't be a huge variance between who is born or dies in the hospital and who gets into the hospital.

Chicago's Department of Health kept the numbers we wanted. The city's longtime health commissioner, Dr. Herman Bundesen, was a cog in the Democratic Machine, which no doubt wanted to downplay any discrimination. But Bundesen, a dedicated public health guy who was both highly respected and popular, maintained considerably more independence than his fellow cogs. As I understood it, he'd struck a bargain with the Machine: the jobs in his department were available to worthy Democratic workers, but if they couldn't cut it, he could, and did, discharge them.

Bundesen had distinguished himself by aggressively helping citizens with TB get the best care. Hoping we could persuade him to give us the "crown jewels" we were seeking, we arranged a meeting. About a half dozen of us met with him in his office and asked for the data: births and death for the previous year by hospital and by race. He listened to our petition, paused for what seemed at the time like a century, but was probably 30 seconds, and said, "All right." And then he pushed the buttons that were necessary to get his staff to bring in the records.

Those records changed the debate. In black-and-white print we saw that in 1953, seventy-one percent of all black hospital deaths occurred at Cook County. Similarly fifty-two percent of all black births took place at County, compared to two percent of the white total. And, as you might imagine, the majority of the non-County hospital births and deaths for black people occurred at black hospitals like Provident.

We published these statistics in a report that was so compelling that a congressman made it part of the *Congressional Record*. More important, in 1955 Chicago's City Council passed the Harvey-Campbell Ordinance. This was not civil rights legislation.

Rather, the law amended existing licensure provisions to prohibit licensed hospitals from denying admission to a patient because of race.

Two years later, we achieved another breakthrough when the City Council enacted legislation to penalize the denial of staff appointments to physicians on the basis of race. These two laws, passed well in advance of the national readiness for civil rights, achieved modest changes in the practices of Chicago's private hospitals. They demonstrated that racism was indeed institutionalized and that the result was literally a matter of life and death. The legislation represented an important statement of public policy and was a harbinger of the historic movement developing nationwide.

In writing about this period I'd be remiss if I didn't relate an experience I had as a member of the AMA. Based on what I've written, you may be surprised to learn I was a member of the AMA. I almost wasn't, but I complained about the organization so much that my senior attendings told me to join and change it from the inside. They also told me the AMA was more democratic than I might imagine.

For better or worse, the AMA had a lot of clout in those days—much more than it does today. It wasn't until about ten years later, in 1965, that the group suffered its first major defeat, when Medicare was passed by Congress over its militant objection.

The AMA was and still is a hierarchical organization that makes it easy for retired doctors, who were and still are really very conservative, to control the apparatus. When I joined, Chicago was divided into some thirteen chapters—an atypical arrangement considering that New York City was simply one big chapter. I attended meetings of the South Side chapter, which had perhaps 1,000 member physicians.

Crohn's Disease was the topic at my first meeting, and there couldn't have been more than seven or eight people in attendance to hear a painful, inept presentation. As I was leaving, the most elderly gentleman in the room approached and said he was delighted to see me and that the brain trust wanted me to run for secretary of the chapter. Secretary, I knew, was a stepping stone to chairman of the chapter, which was a stepping stone to a seat on the Chicago council that represented all the chapters—a big deal.

I was startled. "Sir, you hardly know me."

He nodded, then said, "No, but we have a lot of n——-ers in this branch and we don't want any of them to get elected into office."

Well, that was just the right thing to say to this youthful lefty! I had a decision to make: Respond positively to the offer, or expose the bastard for the racist he was. I accepted the nomination.

Reader, I can see you shaking your head. The story does not end there. I served my term and when it became time for me to move up to chairman, I introduced the person whom I wanted to be the next secretary, the person who would eventually chair the chapter. My choice? My dear African American friend Dr. Clyde Phillips.

Clyde ran for secretary, and his victory effectively ended the unwritten bylaw barring people of color from holding elected office for the AMA in Illinois. Note to the AMA: be careful what you wish for.

My activities to end racial discrimination did not end with this satisfying result. With the Montgomery Bus Boycott of 1956, the civil rights movement began in full force. Leading the effort, of course, was Dr. Martin Luther King, Jr. He became my hero… and my patient.

Five

I would never wish ill health on anyone, certainly not the foremost American civil rights leader of the 20th century and a Nobel Peace Prize winner to boot. Still, I confess that there were times in the mid-1960s when I secretly wished that Dr. Martin Luther King might have had a mild case of the sniffles or some other minor concern that required my attention. As his local physician in Chicago during that period, I treasured the opportunity to talk with him or just bask in his transcendent presence.

The only time that really happened was when the good doctor, who lived for several months on the city's west side in 1966, was laid low—a rarity—and I was summoned to his modest apartment in the heart of the ghetto. Yes, I also marched alongside him to further the cause of the Chicago Freedom Movement and to attend to him in the case of injury. But it's not easy to carry on a conversation when you are ducking bottles, bricks, and rocks.

At the time Dr. King settled into Chicago to fight for open housing and an end to segregation in the public school system, I had known him for about two years. Our first contact took place hundreds of miles to the south—in Mississippi during the Freedom Summer in 1964. He was rising to lead the movement for voting rights, and I was there with other health professionals and volunteers to bear witness and provide medical care to the brave people who were marching, protesting, and sitting-in.

We doctors, nurses, and support personnel were members of a new organization, the Medical Committee for Human Rights (MCHR). I'm proud to say I was an early organizer of this group in Chicago that provided medical service during that summer, during the march from Selma to Montgomery the following year, and at numerous other events to forward the cause of civil rights.

Eventually, we were also involved in the movement to stop the war in Vietnam. Indeed, as I repeatedly told HUAC, I was wearing my MCHR armband in Chicago during the 1968 Democratic Convention.

John Dittmer provides the definitive history of MCHR in his wonderful book, *The Good Doctors*. There is no need to re-tell the story here, but some background is in order. During the late 1950s and early 1960s, progressive doctors in cities across the country worked hard to end discriminatory health care practices. In Chicago, we tried our best through the CEDCMI. Dissatisfied with the AMA's inertia in the movement to end segregation in the medical community, my friend Dr. Bob Smith and fellow activists created the Medical Committee for Civil Rights in 1963. In addition to pressuring the AMA, this group provided care during the March on Washington that year.

MCHR morphed out of this effort the following year as the civil rights movement picked up steam under Dr. King and other leaders. I don't want to leave out names, but among the early organizers and participants were folks like Smith, David French, Arthur Wells, Tom Levin, Alvin Pouissant, Leslie Falk, and June Finer. (June was a brainy, attractive Englishwoman who worked with me at Michael Reese. We dated for a while after Jessie divorced me in 1962. By this time I had five children, Nancy, Polly, Ethan, Barbara and Michael. (Jessie soon married my NU classmate and Cook County roommate, Dr. Tom Sheridan, who had enjoyed many a dinner and evening as our guest.)

Having witnessed the physical abuse that the peaceful protesters endured in places like Birmingham, Alabama—billy clubs, fists, fire hoses, and angry dogs at the hand of law authorities, Klansmen, and "ordinary citizens"—we health professionals knew we would be needed during the Freedom Summer as efforts to register black voters were often met by violence. Sadly, that summer will forever be remembered for the June 21 murders of three dedicated young men who had driven to Neshoba County, Mississippi, to investigate the burning of a black church—James Chaney, Andrew Goodman, and Michael Schwerner.

So when organizers of the Mississippi Summer Project requested medical help, MCHR answered the call. More than 100 of us, mostly from the North, mostly white, headed South that summer and the next. Not all at once, but in shifts, usually of two weeks.

Our numbers included doctors, dentists, nurses, and social workers. Few of us were licensed to practice in Mississippi, a state where an African American's access to adequate health care was as absent as his or her ability to vote. So, we didn't go with the idea of hanging out our shingles.

Our missions were many: Work, in concert when possible with sympathetic local black and a few local white doctors, to better medical care for the disenfranchised; arrange for care and, if need be, hospitalization of sick and injured civil rights workers; and, as a MCHR memo indicated, "above all, provide the presence of sympathetic health personnel in a hostile atmosphere, including visits to jails and participating in civil rights rallies."

In short, we bore not only our doctor's bags, but witness. And what did we see? A familiar pattern. After building community support, the organizers would call for a march followed by a sit-in at a restaurant or bank or store. The authorities would tell them to disperse. They'd refuse. Then the police would arrest them, usually with much more force than was needed, a lot of club swinging. The protesters, mostly, but not exclusively young people, would then be hauled to the local jail and charged with trespassing and violating the local segregation laws.

Pre-arrests, MCHR offered the protesters everyday support— a cup of water, a bandage, first aid. We were, for the most part, immune from police action. Law enforcement made no bones about the fact that they considered us, pardon the phrase, "n----r lovers" who were disrupting the peaceful, wonderful South. Still, they and their fellow white racists had a respect for our profession that was, perhaps, as ingrained as their hatred of black people. While we weren't treated as good friends, we received gentler treatment than the protesters.

Post-police action, our goal was to follow into the jail those arrested. We would ask the authorities if we could go in and visit the prisoners. Invariably they consented. Again, I think it was out of respect for the medical profession. I have no other explanation why they'd want any white interlopers in their prison except that we were *doctors*.

Once in, we would survey each prisoner. If a man or woman behind bars was free from wounds, we would note that loudly. The police understood why we were proclaiming that so-and-so was unhurt when we saw him after the arrest. Because if so-and-so came out of jail battered or bruised, somebody must have roughed him up. This was an effective tactic that diminished jailhouse violence.

It was as a witness, expressing solidarity with those in the movement, that I first saw Dr. King in the flesh. He ran a planning meeting I attended, but he was not running the entire show. Freedom Summer was the brainchild of a quartet of civil rights organizations that included not only King's SCLC, (Southern Christian Leadership Council), but also the Student Non-Violent Coordinating Committee(SNCC), CORE (Congress of Racial Equality), and the NAACP. As a result I met the likes of movement giants like Ralph Abernathy, Stokely Carmichael, James Farmer, and Bob Moses, the intellectual coordinator of the summer who worked so hard for educational opportunities for black kids.

Dr. King and I talked about medical staffing and the do's and don'ts for the doctors on the ground. By this time, he had been in the public eye for almost eight years since leading the Montgomery Bus Boycott. In 1963, he had written his eloquent "Letter from a Birmingham Jail" and he had delivered his dramatic "I Have a Dream" speech at the March on Washington. Here in Mississippi he was, as expected, charismatic, articulate, persuasive, sensible, and modest. He wasn't one to aggressively assert his authority.

We got to know each other very mildly. He had a million things on his plate, but the medical component of the movement was not unimportant. As I observed him over the following years, he seemed to me very collective in his approach. At the same time, he wasn't at all afraid to take unpopular positions.

He was a principled man, as evidenced by his famous speech at the Riverside Church in New York in April of 1967. There, he denounced the Vietnam War, while acknowledging that this stance might turn some of his supporters away from the civil rights movement. "My conscience leaves me no other choice," he said. That is courage.

I went to Mississippi in both 1964 and 1965. Much of my time was spent in the state capital, Jackson—which saw a great deal of violence in '65. Some of my colleagues stayed in the homes of local people. My recollection is that I stayed in motels. The Sun 'N Sand in Jackson rings a bell, although I came for neither sun nor sand... or for the waters.

This was an exhilarating time for most of us. We felt as if we were on the cusp of something very important in the life of our nation. This exhilaration was also fueled by fear or the sense of danger.

When I arrived, I was, to put it mildly, quite naïve. I knew the South was segregated. I knew that blacks were ill-treated. But I didn't have the real day-to-day experience of living inside the civil rights movement and feeling that what happened to Chaney, Goodman, and Schwerner could happen to anyone.

These were violent times. Although I never met a robed Klansman and the worst thing hurled at me were insults, I learned to look over my shoulder and follow certain procedures for safety's sake. Consider these warnings from the MCHR memo:

"Never leave or enter the house in which you are staying when white people are present to observe you. This will meaningfully reduce the probability of reprisals to your hosts.

When leaving the office or hotel, inform someone as to your destination and time of arrival and expected return. If the trip is some distance, call the office when you arrive and again when you leave.

Never leave jail without calling the office.

Make no unnecessary trips, especially at night, and especially not through or in the white community.

Never travel alone (when it is avoidable).

When you travel by car to unfamiliar places, be sure you have adequate instructions, including a map. If you should become lost, ask directions in a Negro community only.

For the rare night travel, the bulb in the ceiling light of your car should be removed to prevent illumination of passengers when car doors are opened."

I wish I'd kept a diary during my stay in Mississippi. I did not, but fortunately Dr. Lee Hoffman, who volunteered in the Clarksdale area, did. Dittmer presents an excerpt in *The Good Doctors*.

"Attended a COFO worker who was beaten over the head. Gave first aid. Accompanied him to the hospital. Played football with local high school boys. Visited several sick local people with nurse. Was arrested for being out after curfew. Visited citizens in jail at request of COFO to give reassurance. I could not have gotten in without positive identification as an MD. Repaired a dangerous electrical connection in a local home. Put a lock on a window in Freedom House. Attended funeral at request of family of a terminal patient I had seen earlier."

I returned to the South with MCHR in March of 1965 and again saw Dr. King. This time he was in Alabama, leading the historic Selma to Montgomery march for a voting rights bill. This was not the March 7 "Bloody Sunday" action that was halted on Day One with tear-gassing and beatings by the police and mounted troopers. (Who can forget the image of the battered John Lewis?) This was the successful five-day trek—often through mud in a cold rain—that was a turning point in the civil rights movement. We escaped the fate of those who had tried two weeks earlier because the whole world was now watching, because President Lyndon Johnson supported the march, and because we were accompanied by some 2,000 National Guardsmen and federal marshals.

With law enforcement present, we MCHR volunteers did not have to attend to "battlefield wounds." We doctored when needed, making sure everyone was well and comfortable. "Everyone" included a lot of dignitaries, many from Hollywood. At night we stayed in churches and other friendly community outposts.

I made an effort to march with many people that week. What

better way to get a sense of who was in the movement, who your allies were. One day I walked alongside a middle-aged white woman. She said she had come because of her religious beliefs. As was typical, local whites howled and hooted at us.

"Why don't these people understand that they've lost their battle? We're all God's children and we should settle this," my new companion lamented.

"True," I said.

But after walking another yards, I turned to her. "Wait a minute," I said. "That's not a simple request you're making of these folks. The black population has been the object of slavery, of rape. Children born of these illicit cohabitations were sold; their own children were sold off as slaves. You're asking a great deal when you're asking them to accept racial equality, because if they do, they plead guilty automatically without a trial to all of these crimes. The only reason that they could get away with it psychologically or legally was to insist on black inferiority. You ask them to forgo that, you ask them to plead guilty to all these evils."

The marches paid off. A version of what came to be known as the Voting Rights Act of 1965 was actually introduced in the U.S. Senate during the period between the Bloody Sunday march and the march that concluded successfully on March 25. Passed by Congress a few months later, it was signed into law by President Johnson on August 6. (Interestingly this was only one week after another piece of Great Society legislation, the act that established Medicare. I will discuss this in the following chapter.)

Officially titled "An act to enforce the fifteenth amendment to the Constitution of the United States, and for other purposes," the Voting Rights Act prohibited states from imposing any "voting qualification or prerequisite to voting, or standard, practice or procedure...to deny or abridge the right of any citizen of the United States to vote on the basis of race or color." No longer could states (read *Southern* states) disenfranchise blacks by requiring them to pass literacy tests or other roadblocks. (Congress has repeatedly renewed and amended the Act over the past 47 years, but as I write this some in government want to terminate the law because they feel it is no longer necessary. Recently the U. S.

Supreme Court struck down Section 4 of the Voting Rights Act, the part of the landmark civil rights law that describes which areas of the country must have changes to their voting laws approved in federal court. I disagree!

We know that most white Mississippians loathed us white Northerners as carpetbaggers. It's fair to ask if there was any resentment of us by the local black community as well. After all, they lived in danger every day just because of the color of their skin. And if they spoke up or joined the movement, the stakes were life and death. As good as our intentions were, we were just passing through for a couple of weeks at a time.

I never felt any animus, but every so often I sensed some in the movement thought we were down there for adventure as opposed to altruism. Eventually MCHR left the South at the behest of local groups who said, in effect, "We're fine. You helped us. Now do something in your own jurisdiction. Chicago, New York you name it, can all do with a little anti-segregation work."

Dr. King realized that the North was the next frontier. Having focused the nation's eyes on the legalized segregation in the South, he wanted to turn attention above the Mason-Dixon line. There, despite the Civil Rights Act of 1964 and the U.S. Supreme Court's 1954 decision in *Brown vs. Board of Education*, de facto segregation was rampant and injurious in education, health care, housing, recreation, and virtually every other aspect of daily life.

In late July of 1965, SCLC launched a five-city "People to People Tour" to pick its city. King's decision later that year to select Chicago was one more example of his savvy and moxie. "The grapes of wrath are stored (in Chicago)," he said.

The city was already the site of one of the most vibrant civil rights efforts in the North. A few years earlier, the Urban League (under Bill Berry), The Woodlawn Organization (under Bishop Arthur Brazier) and the NAACP had enlisted some thirty other local entities from the religious community, union movement, and civil rights movement—of varying degrees of militancy— to form the Coordinating Council of Community Organizations (CCCO). CEDCMI (and later MCHR) was involved from the earliest days, and I attended weekly meetings, most often held in Englewood at

51st and State Street at the YMCA.

CCCO's early target was the Chicago Public School system. Under Superintendent Benjamin Willis, the schools were not only segregated, they were separate and unequal. And Willis showed no willingness to do anything about the sorry state of affairs. African American parents staged sit-ins to do something about overcrowding (the superintendent had cynically brought in buses, dubbed "Willis Wagons" to be used as segregated classrooms). Then, many CCCO members participated in two hugely successful school boycotts that followed the sit-ins—one in October of 1963 and one about four months later. Hundreds of thousands of schoolchildren stayed home.

By the summer of 1965, CCCO, under the leadership of Al Raby, was marching on City Hall and demanding the ouster of Willis. Raby, a young, black schoolteacher was a good man and a good listener. New to such a leadership position, he relied on the counsel of CEDCMI/MCHR for some time.

Enter Dr. King. He was no stranger to Chicago, having spoken to over 55,000 people at a rally at Soldier Field in 1964. Housing as well as education and jobs were to be the focus of what would be called the Chicago Freedom Movement.

When King and his family moved into a $90-a-month, third-floor apartment at 1550 S. Hamlin in the Lawndale neighborhood in January 1966, I had a new patient. Why did he tap me? I didn't ask questions, but I have always assumed it was because we had worked together in the South and I was still part of the movement, now with CCCO. I was an established physician with a reasonably good reputation

My job wasn't so much to take care of his colds or sniffles or broken legs, but to accompany him on his marches when he was very much the target of the local racists. I was supposed to be either to his side or in front of him, physically close. And so I had a front-row seat, albeit a dangerous one, to history. More about the marches shortly.

It's important to note that King did indeed live in the heart of the West Side ghetto, the worst slum in the city. His colleagues—Abernathy and others who joined him for a time in Chicago—

stayed in comfortable hotels and motels. King lived what he believed and preached. His quarters, which also served as movement headquarters, were adequate, but far from sumptuous or elegant.

During King's several month stay in 1966, I was only called to his apartment three or four times. In each instance, the medical issue was minor—a bad cold or the like that might have caused him to take to his bed. He was not a complainer.

If he'd have come to my office, his visit would have lasted 20 or 30 minutes. But I made these calls last all afternoon. His staff would clear out for my examination, so we were alone. And, boy, would I exploit that. He seemed happy to move the conversation from his health to his cause. He never looked at his watch or said, "Shouldn't you be going?"

I've always cherished these encounters, few as they were, as an unusual access to an historic person. Among other things, I remember his observations about money and the black movement. (The way it was pronounced in those days, the accent was on the second syllable. Move*ment* not *move*ment). Dr. King said something to the effect, "Strange thing about our move*ment*: We march and they turn the hoses on us and they put the dogs on us and they club us and people take it. They're courageous, they're disciplined. But if they throw 500 $1 bills in the middle of the room they'll create an endless fight." He was describing how susceptible to corruption these impoverished groups—religious and non-religious—could be.

I put a lot of miles on my feet marching with Dr. King during the summer of '66. On July 10, he gave a speech to over 50,000 people at Soldier Field and then led almost 40,000 on a march to City Hall. There he posted the movement's demands for fair housing, fair employment, and the end to other discriminatory practices.

Weeks later he took the open housing campaign into more hostile territory, the white neighborhoods. On August 5, he led about 700 non-violent protesters into segregated Marquette Park on the Southwest side. We were outnumbered by virulent whites bearing signs that read, "King would look good with a knife in his back." To a popular jingle for Oscar Meyer wieners, some people chanted:

I'd love to be an Alabama trooper
That is what I'd really like to be
For if I were an Alabama trooper
Then I could hang a n----r legally

The *Chicago Tribune* reported:

"As King marched, someone hurled a stone. It struck King on the head. Stunned, he fell to one knee. He stayed on the ground for several seconds. As he rose, aides and bodyguards surrounded him to protect him from the rocks, bottles and firecrackers that rained down on the demonstrators. King was one of 30 people who were injured; the disturbance resulted in 40 arrests. He later explained why he put himself at risk: 'I have to do this—to expose myself—to bring this hate into the open.' He had done that before, but Chicago was different. 'I have seen many demonstrations in the South, but I have never seen anything so hostile and so hateful as I've seen here today,' he said."

I was about two people behind him and was quickly at his side. He endured a large laceration to his head, but was not unconscious. We stopped the blood loss and transported him to the hospital. The event had the capacity to kill him. He was my medical responsibility. In that moment, I was his doctor.

Three weeks later, Dr. King and other leaders from the Chicago Freedom Movement had a summit meeting with Mayor Richard J. Daley. It was announced that the marches would stop and the city would promote fair housing. The agreement did not sit well with more militant blacks who were skeptical of the mayor's sincerity. They proved right.

Mayor Daley went to court and got an injunction preventing future marches in the city. King was critical of the injunction, but obeyed it. There were plenty of suburbs in which housing and employment were also unfair; the marches moved to Chicago Heights and Evergreen Park.

I wish I could say that King's stay in Chicago resulted in immediate, groundbreaking change. Unfortunately, it did not. But if he hadn't started the effort then, who knows how long it would have taken to at least focus attention on the situation and begin the slow march to equality.

I must make one very important point that I don't think is widely known. Nobody doubts that King was very courageous. And they are right.

At the same time, I'm sure vast numbers of people would say he had complete confidence in his cause and its righteousness, that he saw themes of religious and biblical proportion. They are also right.

With this mindset, I'm afraid that the public at large, friend or foe, would also think of him as just ignoring all risk—despite the fact that he ultimately was murdered and that along the way I attended him when he took a rock in the head that split his scalp. They are wrong.

Martin Luther King Jr. was not fearless. When these rocks would be thrown at him, he'd jump. He was very much aware of his own vulnerability. This to me emphatically indicates his courage. He knew of his vulnerability, his mortality, and soldiered on. He was as frightened as anyone would be, but never did that translate into an unwillingness to take a march or to lead the movement.

Six

For better or worse, much of my activity and the activity of MCHR during the 1960s was directly influenced by or in response to the domestic and foreign policies of Lyndon Baines Johnson. Our 36th president did so much to further many of the causes I have believed in for my entire life—civil rights, better access to medical care, early childhood education, the eradication of poverty. But at the same time, he presided over and escalated a deadly, unnecessary war that had devastating consequences at home and abroad for decades. As a result, LBJ will not be placed on a pedestal in these pages. Nor will he be ignored

When, on March 31, 1968, Johnson announced that he would not seek re-election, I was already working to unseat him. The outspoken anti-war Democrat, Senator Eugene McCarthy of Minnesota, was my man. Along with Bill Cousins, the Harvard Law School-educated alderman of Chicago's 8th Ward, I was running in the 3rd Congressional District as a McCarthy delegate to the Democratic convention that would take place in Chicago that August.

Bill, an African American, and I experienced Chicago-style hardball politics up close and personal. The district extended from Hyde Park to the southern border of the city. Back then, as now, most people voted along racial and ethnic lines for "their own." So, in the black neighborhoods, our opponents posted pictures of me; in the white neighborhoods they posted pictures of Bill. As independents, we performed reasonably well, getting about 30 percent of the vote, but we couldn't beat the Machine. Had we won, I guess I would have been inside the convention hall during the convention protests instead of trying to treat the victims of the brutal siege by the Chicago Police.

Providing that medical care is what earned me a ticket to

Washington and a subpoena from HUAC (where Bill Cousins served as my counsel). But before visiting that debacle, let's look at the "good" Lyndon Johnson. His commitment and political savvy gave us, among other things, the Civil Rights Act of 1964, the Voting Rights Act of 1965, and Title XVIII of the Social Security Act. You know this latter provision by its popular name. Medicare. (You may have noticed that I didn't include Medicaid in this list of accomplishments of Johnson's. Medicaid, the health insurance program for the poor enacted in 1965, created health insurance for many of America's poor. But, as the latest variant of the separate but equal doctrine, it proved that a separate program for the poor will always be inferior to a national program that is not based on income.)

I was in active medical practice on July 30, 1965, when Medicare was signed into law by President Johnson. Its impact on older Americans and their families was swift and spectacular. Prior to the signing, only about half of our country's senior citizens had insurance. This wasn't a matter of choice. Most people could only afford coverage through work, and when they stopped working their insurance usually vanished. On a fixed retirement income, few could pay for a policy... if they could even find a company that would insure them.

With Medicare, almost overnight the millions of Americans age 65 and older had the doors to health care opened to them that had hitherto been closed (as did the most severely disabled and those with end stage renal disease). They streamed into our doctors' offices seeking long-deferred and sometimes urgently needed medical attention. Simultaneously, the specter of crushing medical debt was lifted from the shoulders of tens of millions of America's seniors and their families. You could almost hear a collective sigh of relief, though it certainly wasn't coming from the AMA.

Some history: In the late 1950s, some national health insurance advocates in Congress scaled back their dreams of universal coverage and focused on a smaller segment of the population, the elderly. Proposals to pay for the hospital costs of those on Social Security gained traction.

Up to this point, the AMA had never lost a legislative battle. Now, the organization opposed these initiatives just as the National Rifle Association jerks its knee (or trigger finger) every time it perceives that progressive action might reduce its power. Government insurance will most certainly destroy the hallowed doctor/patient relationship, opined the AMA. But surprise, senior citizens and progressives pushed back. In response, the AMA proposed "eldercare"—a voluntary plan that would cover, among other things, doctor services.

After going through the Capitol Hill sausage grinder, Medicare emerged. Financed through Social Security, the plan described in the 133-page bill provided those over 65 with hospital and limited nursing home care, home nursing services and out-patient services. The legislation also created a means for reimbursing doctors for services provided. Called Part B, it paid physicians through a voluntary subsidized system.

On the eve of the signings, the New York *Times* reported, "Earlier today, the president held an unusual meeting lasting nearly two hours with 11 leaders of the American Medical Association, which fought the Medicare bill with every resource at its command." A White House source told the *Times* that LBJ wanted to "convince the doctors that the government was not planning to straightjacket the medical profession." (I will resist the temptation to create my own sentencing regarding the AMA and a straight jacket. The AMA did prevail in its effort to make the program voluntary and to keep the government away from doctors to the extent possible. To wit: "Nothing in this title shall be construed to authorize any federal officer or employee to exercise any supervision or control over the practice of medicine or the manner in which medical services are provided... or to exercise any supervision or control over the administration or operation of any such institution, agency, or person.")

Senior citizens were not the only demographic to benefit from Medicare. The legislation had a direct and positive impact on another one of LBJ's positive initiatives: an end to racial discrimination. How? The Civil Rights Act of 1964 forbade the distribution of federal funds to entities that engaged in segregation.

As a result any institution or organization receiving Medicare funds could not discriminate.

Quentin Young circa 1926 hospitals were at the top of the list of such institutions. If they wanted federal money, they would have to eliminate their long-standing Jim Crow practices. They had until 1966 to change their ways and receive certification from the U.S. Office for Equal Health Opportunity (OEHO). If they didn't comply, they would in all likelihood, be tapped out and out of business.

Not surprisingly, OEHO was understaffed and overwhelmed. Other federal employees were temporarily reassigned to help with certification, but more feet on the ground were needed. A number of civil rights organizations stepped in. Members monitored and even worked at hospitals in the South to insure that certification was warranted and discriminatory practices were eliminated.

This was something to smile about. With us watching and the feds threatening to withhold funds, the hospital floors, waiting rooms, and medical staffs of over 1,000 hospitals were quickly integrated. Signs indicating "white" and "colored" came down. Hospital rooms were desegregated. "Separate but equal" blood supplies for the races were eliminated.

But now a couple of frowns. First, while hospitals had to comply with the provisions of the Civil Rights Act, doctors participating in Medicare did not, said the U.S. Department of Health, Education, and Welfare (HEW, now known as Health and Human Services). Part B was exempted, for what I would argue was no good reason.

A second reason for frowning: As Dr. David Barton Smith, a health policy expert, wrote in a 2005 paper for The Commonwealth Fund: "Since 1968, providers have been insulated from any effective, external Title VI accountability for their federal Medicare and Medicaid funds. The high-water mark of federal health care integration efforts came in 1966. The Office for Equal Health Opportunity was disbanded in 1968 and its Title VI certification responsibilities were shifted to the new, centralized Office for Civil Rights in HEW. For the next critical decade, that office shifted resources to address the issue of school desegregation."

In previous chapters I touched on the failed attempts to enact some kind of national health insurance for Americans of all ages during the presidencies of Franklin Roosevelt and Harry Truman. Of course, I would have preferred a national single-payer system for all under Johnson. Forty-eight years later, I still think such a system is absolutely essential. But at least Medicare was enacted.

Through the years the program has dramatically reduced poverty among the elderly. It added new benefits like preventive care. It reduced racial and income-based disparities. It extended coverage to the severely disabled. It laid the basis for nationwide health studies that have improved the quality of care for everyone. In short, Medicare, a government-sponsored program that now covers over 50 million Americans, has been a triumphant success.

Despite today's whining by the factions that don't want government meddling in our lives, especially with our health care, I haven't encountered too many folks who have burned their Medicare cards in protest. Medicare is, however, facing ominous rumblings from President Obama's debt commission and not-so-veiled threats from other quarters. "Medicare's going broke," its market-obsessed critics say. "It's dragging down the economy."

Such alarms have been sounded about every six or seven years since Medicare's creation, but in real life it continues to thrive. Either the economy prospers, yielding greater tax revenues, or Congress tweaks the payroll tax by a tiny fraction of a percentage point, and immediately the projected shortfall disappears. (The last system-wide adjustment was in 1985, when the rate was increased from 1.30 percent to 1.45 percent.) More progressive taxes are a possible solution as well.

While it is true that aging baby boomers will make bigger demands on Medicare, modest adjustments today will assure its financial solvency tomorrow. In fact, Medicare stands like a rock in a troubled sea of waste, inefficiency and disarray in the rest of our health care system, dominated as the system is by big, corporate insurers whose paramount goal is to maximize profits, achieved by enrolling the healthy, avoiding the sick, raising premiums and denying claims.

Medicare is not without its problems, of course. Its benefits package could be richer. It's been denied the authority to negotiate lower prices with drug companies. The reimbursement rate to physicians could be enhanced and stabilized, instead of depending on an annual cat-and-mouse game with Congress (the "doc fix") over a flawed accounting system that only erodes physician confidence in the program. But the best way to remedy these problems—and to bring down skyrocketing health care costs at the same time—is to improve the program and, most importantly, to expand it to cover every person in the United States. Although the Obama health reform bill, sometimes called Obamacare, does address some of Medicare's problems, its subordination to corporate interests is painfully apparent and precludes uniform success in this country.

That's right: extend Medicare to everyone. By replacing our crazy-quilt, inefficient system of private health insurers with a streamlined, publicly financed single-payer program, we would reap enormous savings. First, we would save about $400 billion annually that is presently wasted on excess paperwork, high salaried executives and costly bureaucracy. That's enough money to cover everyone who is currently uninsured and to upgrade everyone else's coverage without increasing overall U.S. health spending by a single penny. Patients could go to the doctor and hospital of their choice. They'd be covered for all medically necessary services and medications, with no co-pays or deductibles.

Moreover, with Medicare for all, we'd acquire powerful cost-control tools like the ability to purchase medications in bulk, negotiate fees, develop global budgets for hospitals and coordinate capital investments. Such tools would rein in costs and help assure the program's sustainability over the long haul.

Conventional wisdom suggests we should wait and see how the Obama administration's health law plays out. But we've seen how comparable reforms have fared on the state level: they've invariably failed, chiefly because they can't control costs. Meanwhile, more millions suffer and tens of thousands die each year from lack of adequate coverage. Tragically, this picture will not be significantly improved by the new health law. But it's never too late to do the right thing.

**

MCHR, NAACP, and the National Medical Association (NMA) (the alternate to the AMA for black physicians) were among the organizations monitoring the post-Medicare desegregation of the health care system south of the Mason-Dixon Line. The membership of the NMA was almost exclusively black. *Almost*. There were a small number of white doctors, including me.

I've been fortunate enough to meet, treat, and work with a number of remarkable men and women over the years. Some names are familiar to the public. Others are not.

One name that should be is Dr. Leonidas Berry. A 1929 graduate of the University of Chicago Medical School, he wrote several books on his specialty of gastroenterology and even invented a gastroscopic instrument. Indeed, in the 1930s, he was, according to the *New York Times*, "the first doctor to perform gastroscopies, operations involving instruments with which doctors can see inside the digestive tract."

Leonidas conducted much of his research at the University of Chicago, yet never received a deserved faculty appointment from his alma mater… almost certainly because he was black. He was, however, the first black doctor to join the staff of Michael Reese (in 1946) and the first black internist at Cook County Hospital (in 1936). In 1975, when I was chief of medicine at County, he was chief of the endoscopy service.

Active in civil rights in addition to being a groundbreaker, he served as president of the NMA in 1965. I joined that year at his request, eager to show my solidarity and indicate my opposition to the AMA. Black doctors were constantly questioning AMA's racist policies. I felt that I was protesting racial discrimination by joining.

I was more active in MCHR. In April 1965, we gathered at Howard University in Washington, D.C., for our first convention. There we elected Dr. Aaron O. Wells as our first president. An African American from New York City, he had travelled to Mississippi during the Freedom Summer and treated those on the voting rights marches to Selma.

73

At the convention, James Foreman, SNCC's executive secretary, urged us white northerners to work in our own cities. As noted earlier, we did, though many of us also journeyed South again during that summer of '65. I went down to Jackson for a couple of weeks.

Fitzhugh Mullan, a University of Chicago Medical School student whom I count among my close friends, spent the entire summer in Mississippi. As he told an audience at Dartmouth College in 2012, he was put to work, "setting up a health association, doing health education and visiting local doctors and hospitals to raise the issue of segregation, and what we call today huge disparities in health status. 'Medical witness' was a term used in the movement to refer to bringing focus to an issue of indignity or an issue of inequity: visiting doctors offices that had 'colored' and 'white' waiting rooms, hospitals that had segregated wings and the very obvious disparities between the African American population and the white populations."

Meanwhile, MCHR's southern field director, Dr. Alvin Pouissant, was on the ground year-round. Despite a distinguished career in the civil rights movement and as a psychiatrist, Al is probably best known as the adviser to television's groundbreaking *Cosby Show*. Based in Jackson for MCHR, he helped establish and run a community center and health clinic in Tchula, Mississippi, as the organization moved beyond just bearing witness to playing an active role, including lobbying for improvements in public health education and for more and better medical schools that accepted African Americans.

We kept plenty busy up North, too, as the movement became pertinent and at least partially victorious. Those of us living on the South Side of Chicago, where the black population was concentrated, had almost daily evidence of the disparities between the races. There was not as there is today a real middle class of blacks. I remember reading a seminal book on class division within the black community; its author considered postal workers to be the black upper class. Yes, there were exceptions, but in general, through no fault of their own, blacks could not get jobs of managerial leadership. Jim Crow lived in the North as well as the

South, *de facto* if not *de jure*.

In 1967, I became MCHR's third president, its first white one. At the same time we moved our headquarters from New York City to Chicago. I've been asked by several people, how I always seem to wind up as president or chair of a committee or organization. Is it because I like power? Because I'm a control freak? Because nobody else wants to be president?

The short answer is: I don't know. But having said that I'll take a stab. I've lived a long time. I've had a chance to reminisce or ruminate about myself, something all of us do. I think whatever organizational leadership I've demonstrated has its roots in my childhood. Recall, I was double-promoted in grade school—a very bad thing. Getting out of grade school at age 12 and then out of high school at age 16, I had to rely on something other than physical prowess and athletic skill to make my way in my peer group.

The "burden" of leadership didn't bother me. When I went to University of Chicago, I was 16. Some people are quite mature physically at that age. I wasn't. I looked like more like a grade school kid. But if you wanted to be a leader in a student political organization, there was no requirement that you had to look like a mature, middle-aged person. If you were willing to give it the time, you could have a leadership role. That happened successively as time went on. And by the end of my U. of C. stint, I was 18 and was actually treated like a normal human being.

And there's this: I always loved a battle. Still do. I've never tired of the good fight. And with respect to civil rights circa 1967 and MCHR, the good fight was needed from Mississippi to Chicago and everywhere else. The stakes were too high to ignore. I enlisted, but I certainly wasn't the only one.

The membership of MCHR had varying opinions on what issues we should and should not get involved in. As President Johnson escalated the war in Vietnam some in our organization wanted us to oppose the conflict and call for withdrawal from military activity in Asia. There was good reason to oppose. The United States went from about 15,000 "military advisers" in Vietnam in 1963 to over half a million troops in five years. U.S. casualties?

58,000 deaths and 300,000 wounded. That's not counting the hundreds of thousands of South Vietnamese and North Vietnamese soldiers and civilians, and those in the neighboring countries.

Led by a charismatic Californian named Bill Bronston, the younger members of MCHR, medical students in particular, argued that the organization's silence on the war was antithetical to our mission to eliminate segregation. They cited the disparity between the draft status of young white and black men. Many whites had the means to keep themselves out of service. Not so the blacks.

I didn't disagree with the facts, but initially I did disagree with the tactics. We were all against the war, of course, and each of us could point to the various anti-war movements to which we belonged. But many of us believed it was not fair for us as an adjunct to the black movement to create a problem for it by taking an organizational stance against the war.

We weren't the only ones facing this "should we or shouldn't we?" debate. It's fair to say that many of the more conservative black ministers in the civil rights movement didn't want these two issues melded. They were at long last getting some leverage on segregation. They didn't want to go down as kind of an anti-war sidebar that alienated their mainstream supporters.

Dr. King finally put that to rest with that glorious speech at the Riverside Church.

At our 1965 convention the students' anti-war resolutions were defeated. By spring of 1967, however, with the war having escalated even further, we were ready to take a stand. We passed a resolution calling for "unilateral, immediate cessation of hostilities." Later I received a letter from Dr. King in which he said he was "especially happy" with MCHR's public position. "We must continue to raise our voices loudly and clearly to end this tragic war," he wrote. Toward that end, MCHR and other anti-war medical groups created COHO, the Council of Health Organizations.

As Dittmer writes in *The Good Doctors*, "In addition to its public position, MCHR became more directly involved when it initiated a program to provide physical examinations for young men facing the draft." Psychiatrists also participated. This wasn't a far-fetched venture. The fact was, until a lottery system was instituted in 1968, it was easy to stay out of the service if you stayed in school—in other words if you were a white person of means. Blacks and the working poor were far less likely to do so.

While an examination by a private physician or psychiatrist was not legally dispositive, many draft boards relied on such exams in determining whether a young man was physically and psychologically capable of service. Of course as doctors we were obliged to be honest in our evaluations. Our principal service was just making ourselves available to young men who otherwise would not have been able to see a doctor who could identify a condition that might legitimately prevent military service. Common exclusionary findings included allergies, vision defects, and hearing impairments.

We had a rule: When a white patient came, he also had to bring a black patient with him in order to receive the service. We were in about twenty cities. SNCC and CORE and ministers helped get the word out. We didn't have to set up additional clinic hours for the initiative; it was integrated into routine care. For some young men, this was the first time they had seen a provider since they were born. We tried to make our services available to people in the ghettos and the barrios. We were worried about being inundated, though we were not faced with that challenge.

The doctors were very strict. We didn't play fast and loose with the rules; the young people had the maladies that were reported. Our goal was to level the playing field, giving young people with limited or no medical history this service and a fair physical exam.

**

The remainder of this chapter might be titled, *A Tale of Two Cities*. The cities? Washington, D.C. and Chicago. The year 1968.

We begin in the spring. Dr. King and his Poor Peoples' Campaign (PPC) were scheduled to arrive in the nation's capital in April to demand better services for the poor and disenfranchised. They planned to stay a while in a tent city.

King appealed to the medical community for assistance, and MCHR agreed to provide care for those who assembled. Months before the scheduled arrival of the protesters, MCHR began talking with local health and law enforcement officials. Everyone was aware that in the wake of racial turbulence in other cities, violence was possible. After assuring these officials that its mission was medical not political, MCHR, as Dittmer notes, "received permission from the police to visit inmates in jails and from local hospitals to coordinate activities in case of emergency."

Tragically, King was assassinated in Memphis on April 4. This was a tremendous blow to the movement. It was particularly brutal because he was young and had so much promise for not only the nation, but the world. Along with millions of others, I was deeply demoralized. We wondered then whether there was any hope of escaping the evils of racism.

The assassination triggered riots in cities from coast to coast, including Washington. After three days and nights, twelve people were dead, hundreds were injured, and over 7,500 were arrested. In an ideal world, MCHR would have worked in concert with the police and the local medical institutions. And that's pretty much what happened. Ten police precincts appealed to us for help in treating prisoners, and forty of our doctors responded. On the street, one of our doctors saved the life of a soldier who'd had a heart attack during the riots.

When the PPC arrived in mid May, MCHR joined the NMA and others to provide care to the shantytown known as Resurrection City. Dittmer writes that, "Relations between the two national organizations had always been problematic." By this I suppose he means that the NMA focused on physician opportunities/prerogatives, while the medical communities had an enlarged agenda.

Dittmer goes on to say, "MCHR chair Quentin Young went out of his way to appear cooperative and non-threatening." He cites a letter I sent to NMA chairman Lionel Swan in which I expressed "our willingness to collaborate with all concerned medical groups, especially NMA."

**

From cooperation to chaos. The story of the clashes between police and protesters during the Democratic convention in Chicago is well known. Several thousand protesters descended on Chicago during the last week of August 1968. For the most part, they came to register their opposition to the war… peacefully, if not quietly.

Movement leaders were outspoken. Their language was confrontational, even offensive to some who agreed with their cause. But encouraging civil disobedience in the face of an intransigent city that refused to give permits to assemble and speak is far different from encouraging violence. The protesters were not armed with billy clubs; they didn't carry tear gas or mace. They had no marching orders to bang heads. And they were outnumbered by the police and National Guard. There were about 10,000 demonstrators compared with over 20,000 police and National Guard.

Tensions between the protesters and the police simmered for several days, regularly spilling over into physical confrontation. On Sunday, August 25, police forcibly removed a crowd attempting to sleep in Lincoln Park on the near North Side. Billy clubs and tear gas were the weapons du jour. Reporters as well as protesters were injured.

The most infamous clash took place three days later. On the 28th, while "the whole world was watching," a riot broke out. A police riot. Protesters attempting to march down Michigan Avenue to the convention at the International Amphitheatre were clubbed and gassed, bloodied and beaten. Some policemen were also injured as the protesters responded to the attack.

Much of the action took place right outside the Hilton Hotel, where the Democratic nominee for president, Vice President Hubert Humphrey, was staying. On the convention floor, Connecticut Senator Abraham Ribicoff denounced the police action. Mayor Richard J. Daley mouthed x-rated epithets that most agree included anti-Semitic slurs directed at the Jewish Ribicoff.

Along with many others from MCHR, I was in the thick of the battle. Soon after the Democrats announced in the fall of 1967 that the convention would be held in Chicago, MOBE (the National Mobilization Committee to End the War in Vietnam) contacted us. Would we provide medical care to the protesters if and when? Of course.

MOBE told us hundreds of thousands of demonstrators would be coming to Chicago. Though the actual numbers never approached that, we had no reason to contest these figures. We weren't in the business of making estimates. We were asked to provide a medical presence much as we did in the South. With several years of experience in these matters under our lab coats, we knew what to do.

MCHR always made it clear that it would not interfere with existing institutions that provided medical care. And so our first move—many months before the convention—was to make overtures to all the public agencies that were responsible for maintaining order and giving help, medical and otherwise, where needed. Topping the list were the Chicago Department of Health, the police department, and the fire department.

We soon saw a pattern emerging. Initially, we would have a positive meeting with a decision-maker in a department—the head of public health or the fire department, for example. Already there was an awareness that this was not going to be your run-of-the-mill convention. We noted that we were volunteers with much experience in the South. We didn't expect the hostility from the police that the demonstrators had experienced. We just wanted to collaborate with the city in any way it wanted. We didn't expect beatings. We expected casualties from heat stroke, exhaustion, or accidents. When large numbers convene, people fall ill or get hurt.

At these early powwows, we were treated nicely—as citizens should be treated by their government. But when we'd come back to start getting down to specifics, the dynamic was dramatically different. Word must have come down not to cooperate with us. It became clear that we were not going to have any collaboration with official agencies. Not in Richard J. Daley's Chicago. That was not only disappointing, it was frightening. Remember, most everyone was expecting close to half a million protesters.

Cut off from the city, we did what we could do through our modest, albeit real, resources in the Chicago area. We undertook a general mobilization of professional people to meet whatever health and medical problems arose. We asked volunteers to sign up to be available for a certain number of hours on one or more

days. We also identified about a dozen venues—mostly churches—that would receive casualties. Again, at this point, "casualties" meant those with heat stroke or a twisted ankle. This was
Chicago, after all, not Selma.

We made some progress. Many MCHR members worked at
or with local medical schools or hospitals. They signed up fellow
professionals, though far from the number needed to deal with the
estimated number of demonstrators. We had something going, but
not anything that could handle the problems that half a million
people might experience.

In the months before the convention, we also met with
people from the movement. This movement didn't have a single
identifiable leader. It was more of a coalition—a friendly coalition, it appeared to us. We explained to these folks what resources
we had—a dozen or so first aid centers and maybe 40 volunteer
health care professionals.

Here I must speak about my friend and Chicago chapter co-
chair Jane Kennedy. She was a skilled nurse, devoted to the anti-
racism movement. Jane joined a Catholic anti-war group, Beaver
55, and they destroyed the files of those that were on the draft list.
Eventually they were caught and she went to jail. They were very
heroic. I visited her when she was jailed. Unfortunately, she got
very depressed while incarcerated.

MCHR was not the most important element in the anticipated activities, numerically or otherwise. But we weren't unimportant. We attended some of the planning meetings, and we
told the organizers what we had and, equally important, what we
hoped to see happen. Recognizing that they couldn't control all
who assembled, we asked that they tell people to be orderly and
not panic. We weren't expecting a police riot, but we were aware
that Mr. Daley and his minions were not doing much to ensure
there would be a nice, orderly, peaceful demonstration. City Hall
denied almost every MOBE request for a permit to march or assemble.

As we will see in the next chapter, HUAC made a big deal of
the fact that I met with one of MOBE's leaders, Rennie Davis, in
the spring of 1968 and then lent him some money so that he could

rent office space used for protest planning. I knew Rennie because of his work in Chicago's Uptown neighborhood, where he was doing community organizing to assist those migrating from Appalachia.

I also knew Rennie, as well as many others, because of our mutual commitment to the "peace movement." I had been doctor for Students for a Democratic Society (SDS) some years earlier when it was a peaceful, joyous, non-violent outfit with an inspiring libertarian notion of social reform. To my dismay, in subsequent years it changed its character rather quickly—a good, if sad, example of the impatience of young people when they want social change. There's no doubt in my mind that the dalliance with violence elected Mr. Nixon in 1968, to put it bluntly.

To most of the leaders in organizations like SDS or MOBE, I was an old-timer, twenty years their senior. But my medical skill gave me an entree to these younger people that I wouldn't otherwise have had. I don't mean they would have barred me at the door, but they had their own optimistic view that their generation was going to rescue the world, America included. And folks like me with twenty years or more of left-wing identification? Well, we were nice people, but we had it wrong. We didn't realize what the real answer, in the opinion of many of them, was: militancy.

So what did the decidedly non-militant MCHR do when the protesters arrived in town? We proceeded to Lincoln Park, where, as noted, the police used excessive force to remove about 1,000 people who refused to respect the 11 p.m. curfew. At the beginning we had several church-sponsored emergency care centers around the periphery of the Loop. We had doctors and nurses stationed to give first aid as needed. I used to go around to the centers and make sure they were protected and active. It got progressively worse.

As word spread about the police action that Sunday night, something remarkable happened. Doctors and other health care workers phoned our office and enlisted. Over the next day or two, our numbers increased dramatically—up close to 500. As Dittmer notes, "The volunteers, easily identifiable in their medical attire, were also forcibly ejected from Lincoln Park each night, despite an earlier agreement with the city that medical workers would be regarded as 'neutrals' and given access to the wounded."

On Wednesday night, when the full-scale riot broke out, we were transformed into battlefield medics. Some people were injured. Most wounds were inflicted on the neck and back or the head. Protesters were struck as they fled. I was active in providing first aid and continued to go to the different centers to make sure the staffing and supplies were adequate.

To no one's surprise, Mayor Daley saw the events differently than the participants, the press, and the millions of television viewers who watched in horror as the police went wild. His report, titled *The Strategy of Confrontation*, blamed outside agitators ("revolutionaries" and "terrorists") who came to the city looking for a fight.

According to this post-mortem, "It appeared (to the casual reader) that more than three times as many police (198) had been injured as demonstrators (60)," Dittmer writes. He goes on to note that about half of the injuries sustained by the police were either self-inflicted (tear gas) or insignificant.

Daley's inaccurate, offensive report demanded a response. A few days later, I led an MCHR press conference at which we presented that response. Our report, *The Strategy of Contusion,* set the record straight. Again, thanks to John Dittmer for the following summary:

"The Medical Committee had written records on 425 protesters treated at the 'stationary medical centers.' Of these 112 suffered from head, face, or neck wounds, 83 had injuries to the body or below the neck, and more than 80 were treated for the effects of tear gas and mace. Mobile medical teams, unable to keep records, reported treating an additional 200 to 300 people for medical conditions and provided first aid for tear gas and mace to another 400 to 600 demonstrators. The MCHR report projected about a thousand casualties, with both hard and empirical evidence to back it up."

In retrospect, the scene in Chicago brought great credit to MCHR. While we have records of over 1,000 patients, undoubtedly there were many more that sought care from area hospitals and facilities. Many people received care apart from the MCHR activities, but by and large the conduct of our volunteers was orderly and laudable.

Unfortunately, both confrontation and contusion continued in the months that followed. Chicago saw a kangaroo court, while Washington saw a kangaroo congressional committee. I was called to testify before each of them.

Seven

Mr. Smith (counsel to HUAC): Dr. Young, are you a member of the Communist Party?

Dr. Young: Sir, apparently you did not hear my earlier statement or you wouldn't have bothered to ask me that question. It is perfectly clear that that question is irrelevant to anything that happened in Chicago during the week in question. It is also further clear that I could answer that question without any embarrassment. But I would not compromise the rights of all Americans by responding to such an obvious violation of the First Amendment privileges and the variety of others I have cited. You may relax on that one.

Recently a friend likened my appearance in front of HUAC in October 1968 to a Groucho Marx performance. This was a new take on an old, but memorable milestone. I thought for a moment. Groucho Marx? The master of orchestrated anarchy? A fellow whose repartee confused and undressed windbags and the self-important? I turned to my friend and said, "Thank you."

In this chapter, I'll tell the story of my appearance before a committee of old, self-important windbags who had the power to throw me into jail. I will also tell the story of my involvement in a second proceeding that was spawned by the events outside the convention hall in Chicago. The trial of the Chicago Seven (originally there were eight), which began in September 1969, saw prominent anti-war activists charged with, among other things, conspiracy and inciting a riot. I was not one of the defendants, but did play a fairly well-publicized, if minor, role as the doctor who gave Abbie Hoffman the stay-home-from-court permission slip.

What can be said about the House Un-American Activities Committee? Here's what I said when afforded the opportunity to make an opening statement on October 3, 1968. "Mr. Chairman, I wish to inform you that on October 2nd I instructed my counsel to enter a suit in Federal Court reflecting my belief that the Committee is now and has been an illegal and unconstitutional tribunal."

I'd been following the heinous activities of the Committee since the late 1930s when it had a slightly different name— House Committee on Un-American Activities—but the same mission. Under the leadership of Congressman Martin Dies, it tried to block many of FDR's progressive programs, while also searching out so-called subversives. (Interestingly, its enemies list did not include the virulent Ku Klux Klan. One committee member said, "The threats and intimidations of the Klan are an old American custom, like illegal whiskey making.")

Over the years HUAC destroyed the lives of hundreds if not thousands of good Americans, most famously during its 1947 investigation of the motion picture industry. From Hollywood to the halls of academia, many men and women lost their reputations and livelihoods thanks to the Committee. Some were even driven to suicide.

HUAC was on the prowl—as was a federal grand jury— within days of the convention's end. Why? The Committee wanted to investigate published rumors that Communists had fomented the riots in Chicago. The hearings were titled, "Subversive Involvement in Disruption of 1968 Democratic Party National Convention."

In my opinion, however, there was more here than met the eye. There is little doubt in my mind that Mayor Daley, who had considerable clout with the majority Democratic U.S. Congress, was behind this. Whether he chose to acknowledge it or not, he and his well-run Machine had been embarrassed by the events of late August—events which were later characterized as a "police riot" in the independent Walker Report.

It's one thing when your police beat up demonstrators. It's quite another when they clobber the press, literally. Several reporters were beaten with fists or clubs. Those are Nazi Germany tactics.

The Fourth Estate fought back with words and pictures—the truth—and in so doing created a huge public relations disaster for the city. Hizzoner, I believe, wanted vindication from Congress. And HUAC, which had gradually lost its clout and was now seen as a largely irrelevant adjunct of the right-wing extremists, saw an opportunity to be relevant again. (During the Vietnam era, the Committee had tried to hold hearings around the country. The protests were so powerful that HUAC retreated to Washington and never ventured beyond the Beltway again.)

And so, a last gasp witch hunt was in order.

Who were the witches? The Committee subpoenaed the usual suspects, including Yippies Abbie Hoffman and Jerry Rubin and fellow anti-war activists Rennie Davis and David Dellinger. If my verbal jousting called to mind Groucho Marx, then perhaps Rubin and Hoffman called to mind another Marx brother. The Yippies weren't silent like Harpo—they never were—but they utilized props to great effect—draping themselves in the American flag and the flag of the Viet Cong. Rubin even showed up dressed as Santa Claus.

For the record, I wore a suit and tie. And while the antics of my fellow witnesses were amusing to some, I found it hard to laugh. First, as I would later say on the record, the Committee had a thirty-year hallmark of "constitutional violations, character defamations, and the chilling effect on guaranteed liberty." And on a personal level, we all faced a harsh reality: this Committee, no matter how irrelevant or unconstitutional we might deem it, still had the power to hold any of us in contempt. That, or proof of perjury, could lead to jail time.

As I was not a usual suspect, I was surprised to receive the subpoena. I hadn't crossed state lines to organize a demonstration. I hadn't even demonstrated. I'd merely given medical assistance to the demonstrators—and as I told the Committee, to the injured police as well.

So why was HUAC interested in me? Well, there was the fact that the Chicago chapter of MCHR, of which I was the head, had participated in planning meetings with MOBE before the convention. There was the fact that I had loaned Rennie Davis $1,000, which was apparently used to rent space for MOBE. And there was my inglorious past, replete with rumored associations that made the mouths of the HUAC bulldogs water.

The Committee asked about my association with this subversive group or that one thirty years earlier. And what about the fact that I had signed a "friend of the Court" brief in support of the Communist Party's constitutional challenge of the Subversive Activities Control Act?

Seriously? I had put my name on a Supreme Court brief. I did not know that was worthy of congressional scrutiny.

While I refused to answer the Committee's questions about my affiliation with the Communist Party, I had no trouble answering the same question outside the hearings when the press asked. The answer was, No.

My subpoena arrived on September 23, giving me less than 10 days to prepare. First stop? My lawyer, Ira Kipnis. An astute professional, he told me I could take the Fifth Amendment and that would be the end of it.

"I can't take the Fifth," I said.

"Why?"

I explained that I was being subpoenaed to describe the activities, or, more accurately, condemn the activities of the Medical Committee in supplying medical support to the people who were protesting at the Chicago convention. While I loved the Fifth Amendment and had no hesitancy in invoking it as part of my constitutional rights, I had a concern:

Four hundred health professionals had volunteered during the convention. What would I do when HUAC asked me if Dr. X., whom I may not even know, is a member of the Communist Party. If I invoke the Fifth, X is all of a sudden under a cloud of suspicion. Remember, you can't invoke the Fifth selectively to answer particular questions; it's all or nothing.

I presented an alternative to Ira: refuse to answer certain questions because they violated my First Amendment rights of Free Speech. He didn't begrudge me that position. At the same time, however, he did his duty by informing me that he thought

I was being foolhardy; the courts had previously ruled that the First Amendment does not offer the same protection as the Fifth. I could be held in contempt by refusing to answer based on the First Amendment.

"If I use the First Amendment defense and they find me in contempt, what's the penalty?" I asked.

"A year in jail."

"If I do that twelve times, is that twelve years?"

"No. They're concurrent."

If Ira had said that invoking the First Amendment one hundred times would get me 100 years in jail, I might have thought twice. But with a maximum of one year? *Hell*, I thought. *I've been told federal prison is better than state prison. And I'm a doctor, so maybe they'll assign me to the medical wing.* All this to say that I wasn't apprehensive. I knew what the consequences were, and I was willing to take them.

Step Two, no offense to Ira, was to ask the ACLU for help. I had a long association with the group, serving on the Chicago board for many years, and knew it had a marvelous record of opposing the Committee. I was delighted when Jeremiah Gutman, who was based in New York, was assigned to represent me. He was a lawyer in private practice, but he had been before HUAC many times as counsel for people who were subpoenaed.

Gutman was a helluva bright guy, somewhat colorful in his own right. Here's how the *Village Voice* described him: "an ACLU-type lawyer with a Talmudic beard and a necktie of many colors that can only have been bought for him by his wife."

The Committee rules were quite different from a courtroom or any reasonable hearing. A witness was allowed to have counsel present, but the lawyer was not supposed to participate in the hearing. He or she was there for the witness to turn to and ask advice. But he/she was not permitted to object to anything.

Gutman, like the best lawyers in these venues, was bold. He pushed the envelope—even leaving himself open to charges of contempt. I quickly picked up on the fact that I could take a cue from his remarks to the chair. He'd speak out in anguish about the question or the way they were treating me. In turn, I'd repeat those things that he had said. I don't mean to say that I had nothing to offer, but I was guided by a very skilled lawyer in that Congressional hearing.

On the eve of my appearance, we witnesses and our lawyers met in a hotel room. Those lawyers included my friend Bill Cousins, who had asked if he could assist with my representation, and the renowned Bill Kunstler.

Also present were several friends of the other witnesses, including Paul Krasner, another prominent anti-war Yippie, who was editor of the humorous left-wing *Realist* magazine. One of the lawyers noted that if these friends remained in the room, the Committee could subpoena them and ask what had transpired. And our lawyers could also be questioned because they weren't speaking to us privately. Our speech would no longer be protected by the attorney-client privilege.

The lawyers went around the room and asked us if we wanted the friends to stay. Hoffman and Rubin and some others said to let them stay for our briefing; there was nothing to hide. Dellinger, older and more mature, was wary.

And me? I had no intention of compromising the attorney-client privilege.

"Get them the hell out of here!" I said. I wanted every protection I could get. All I needed was to have Krasner or one of the lawyers subpoenaed and asked, "What did Dr. Young say there?"

It's idiocy to have your private communications open to review by your opponents. I wasn't going to grovel before the Committee. But on the other hand, I wasn't going to give them access to privileged information.

That same evening, Gutman told me, "I want you to write a statement."

"Fine," I said. "What should I put in it?"

"Put what you want to say," he said handing me pen and paper.

My opening statement read in part: "Certain of the unconstitutionality of this tribunal, I would not be a party to its hearings. However, since the Medical Committee for Human Rights played such an exceptionally courageous and humane role during convention week and since city officials of Chicago and more recently police officers of Chicago have sought to besmirch this record of unselfish service, I must tell the American people the truth of our Medical Committee's actions."

**

The hearing room was full. People lined up to wait for seats. As expected, the atmosphere was somewhat circus-like. Rubin and Hoffman were more distracting than disruptive. At one point Committee chair Richard Ichord told them that if they wanted to smoke, they would have to go outside.

There was an air of levity, but I don't want to diminish the gravity of the hearing. The Committee had investigators who had been out in the field doing their homework. They produced witnesses, mainly police spies who had posed as friends of the protesters but were really informing on them.

The hearing was aimed at discrediting the protesters and, by implication, the medical work. My testimony was an attempt to give a different picture of it. I did this by talking about MCHR's role in the Selma march and other momentous events and by citing a letter from the District of Columbia police praising our efforts during the riots there. As for Chicago, I noted that we had records of over 1,000 people who had some kind of medical need that we took care of.

I wasn't particularly pleased by the behavior of Hoffman and Rubin. HUAC deserved to be mocked, but I'm not sure in the battle for the hearts and minds of America that parody was the best strategy.

I took my strength during this period from my outrage at the Committee, my belief in MCHR, and from friends and others in the movement and medical community who provided moral support, privately and publicly. Before I headed east, friends gathered to wish me luck. In D.C., Fitzhugh Mullan and others visited. The Student American Medical Association, normally a conservative group subordinate to the AMA (which remained silent), made statements on my behalf. The Student Health Organization and an association of health students also rallied support. MCHR, of course, was also behind me. I felt neither alone nor a victim.

I don't think the HUAC congressmen and staff ever figured me out. I dressed differently than most of the other witnesses, I didn't try and turn the hearing room into a theatre, and I was a doctor. Still, I was somewhat the hostile witness. I demanded apologies from the chair for his insults and invoked my supposedly non-existent First Amendment rights on numerous occasions. The chair repeatedly told me I could be held in contempt, but he never pulled the trigger.

If you look at the testimony, you'll see that I began on the defensive. The Committee sparred with me, suggested I was somehow supportive of violence, alleged I had been a member of the Communist Party. But by the end, I think they just sort of gave up. I read from *The Strategy of Contusion*. They couldn't get the goods on me because there were no goods to get.

The strategy of the committee was clear. They had police testimony I gave $1,000 to Davis, attended MOBE meetings, donated money to the anti-war movement. Which of those would you say is un-American? I pushed back.

"Mr. Smith: Information has been furnished to the committee by a confidential source that the cards in the Office of the National Mobilization Committee contained the name of Dr. Quentin Young, M.D., with his home address, telephone numbers, and contained notes as follows:

Mr. Cousins: Mr. Chairman, we want to inspect what he is going to read from.

Mr. Gutman: We are getting unsworn testimony in violation of the Fourth Amendment, I presume.

Dr. Young: If you will hear me—sir, will you hear me?

Mr. Ichord: I am trying to get the question put and then I will rule. You are not permitting the question to be put.

Dr. Young: Mr. Ichord, you have been extremely fair. Listen carefully.

Mr. Ichord: I am trying to be.

Dr. Young: If I am going to be defamed by this ridiculous

stuff, it is on your head. Sir, it is on your head. It is on your head! Read it and make sure that if that can't be cross-examined, I will not be defamed. Do you want that publicly stated. Do you want to defame me?"

Mr. Ichord: Rephrase your question, Counsel.

Mr. Smith: Are you aware that your name was in the files of the National Mobilization Committee to receive invitations, receive mail, to receive funding requests, and that you were noted as a primary contact of MCHR.

Dr. Young: No.

Mr. Smith: Did you ever make a contribution to the National Mobilization Committee in the sum of a $125 check?

Dr. Young: Sir, I can't recall that, but I would not deny that I made that. I have made many contributions... I find this a shameful invasion of my right to donate money."

When the chairman told me I was excused, I told him I wasn't finished yet. HUAC was, however. It died shortly after these hearings.

**

A UPI story, December 26, 1969, reported: "U.S District Court Judge Julius J. Hoffman was to rule on whether the trial should continue in the absence of one of the defendants Abbie Hoffman. The Yippie leader was hospitalized for bronchial pneumonia his attorneys said. Abbie Hoffman was not in court Wednesday. His attorney Leonard Weinglass told Judge Hoffman that his client refused to waive his rights to be at each session of the trial. Hoffman had been on the witness stand and had not finished his testimony when his illness was announced. The judge put Hoffman's doctor, Dr. Quentin Young, on the stand to testify about his condition. The doctor said X-rays of Hoffman's lungs showed several abnormalities. He said Hoffman should stay in bed for four or five days at Michael Reese Hospital. At the request of the prosecution Dr. Joseph Freilich of the department of thoracic medicine at St Joseph's Hospital was to examine Hoffman and report his findings to the court."

Of course the HUAC hearings did not spell the end of the federal government's attempts to hold the convention demonstrators responsible for the violence on the street during the convention. A grand jury eventually indicted eight activists for conspiracy and inciting riots. In addition to Hoffman, Rubin, Davis, and Dellinger, we now had Tom Hayden, Bobby Seale, Lee Weiner, and John Froines. The Chicago Eight would soon become the Chicago Seven when the imperious Judge Julius Hoffman severed Seale from the case for what is best described as "conduct unbecoming." The Black Panther leader had created a ruckus in the courtroom by insisting he was entitled to a lawyer of his own choosing. Showing no judicial restraint, the judge had ordered him restrained —bound and gagged to be precise—before banishing him.

The tale of the trial—a frame-up in my opinion—has been well told by journalists and historians. I was merely a footnote. But sometimes footnotes make for entertaining, if not insightful stories. So I will tell you mine.

It begins in December 1969. By that time the trial had been playing for three months. I use that word "playing" on purpose. What took place in the courtroom was closer to theatre than a legal proceeding. Theatre from the bench. And theatre from the defense table.

But if the goings-on in the courtroom were surreal, the goings-on in the streets were all too real. Protesters regularly made their feelings known outside the federal court building. The demonstrations were generally without incident... until the second week in October. Beginning October 8, the Weathermen faction of SDS began its "National Action," built around a new strategy: "Bring the war home."

By Saturday, October 11, that war was being waged in the Loop and on Michigan Avenue, as about 300 demonstrators broke through police lines and started smashing windows of stores and cars. In the melee, a lawyer for the City of Chicago was permanently paralyzed while trying to subdue one of the protesters. We now refer to these doings as the Days of Rage.

I was a mere spectator of the trial from afar until just before

Christmas. My bit part began when I got a late evening phone call at home from Leonard Weinglass, a terrific lawyer, who along with Kunstler was representing the defendants. To the best of my recollection, our conversation went something like this:

"Quentin," Weinglass said, "Abbie is sick and I wonder if you can see him."

"Sure. I'll make him my first patient in the morning."

Then the kicker. "Well, he's on the stand, and it would be good if we could get an evaluation. The judge is very hostile."

"Yeah."

"It's respiratory."

Always at the service of these ideologues, I said, "Why don't you take him to Michael Reese. I'll call ahead and make sure he gets a chest x-ray and I'll join you in a half hour when the film will be ready to read and we have something going."

As planned, I appeared later that evening and found Weinglass with a sullen Hoffman, who was coughing. I looked at the x-ray. "Not very much there. Maybe in the corner there's some fluid. Looks like it's a bronchial infection."

I turned to Weinglass. "I'll give him medicine. He should be good in two or three days."

"Well, the problem is he's on the stand. It's already a show. The last thing Judge Hoffman would want is for us to interrupt the trial with a cold. "

"Well, tell the judge he'll be okay in a day or two."

"Nah, they can't do it like that. He's on the stand."

I was beginning to get the picture. Weinglass didn't tell me what to do, but he hinted strongly. "Well," I said, "if it's a question of him being on the stand in this condition or being treated, I'll hospitalize him for a day or two."

Weinglass was savvy. "Don't do anything just to help us. Do whatever you think is right."

Boy was I naïve. It took me a long time to realize that Hoffman wasn't ready for his testimony. He'd been a bad witness up to that point and they needed a reason to keep him off for a while. And now he wasn't going to show up because I said he should be hospitalized.

I woke up the next morning and drove to the hospital to make my rounds. On my way, I was, in effect, subpoenaed by radio. "And Judge Hoffman has insisted that Dr. Young appear in court with the X-rays... "

Oh my. I started thinking that some of my many, shall we say, unfriendly colleagues might relish the opportunity to come to court and dispute my diagnosis of Abbie Hoffman's condition. They might even go so far as to suggest I was trying to screw up the justice system by concluding Hoffman needed to be hospitalized.

When I got to Reese, I was greeted by a slew of people on the staff. Slowly, too slowly, I was becoming aware that this was no fun and games. This was the real thing.

Someone said, "Dr. So-and-so wants you to call him immediately. Here's the number."

The doctor turned out to be a lawyer, not a doctor. Weinglass. I learned subsequently that his phone—the defense's private line—was tapped. "Quentin," he said, "there's nothing to worry about. Just bring the x-ray and we'll talk about what the process is."

"I'm not worried," I said, "but as you talk I get increasingly so."

"Go see your patient, so you can report the latest from the front."

Hoffman had a private room in the fancy part of Michael Reese. And in that room, there were two or three girls, including one in bed with him. (Much as I think government should assume the cost of patient care, I do not think the girls qualified as a reasonable expense.)

My patient was not only canoodling, he was smoking. I could sense the peril moving from him to me.

I got the latest X-rays and talked to him. He had a slight cough. He was smart-alecky. What's new? This was a guy who was wearing judicial robes to court and calling the judge his long -lost father. That shtick does not in the long run effect change.

Due to take the stand in the courtroom of the other Hoffman at 10 a.m., I rushed downtown for a quick briefing with Weinglass. He told me he'd be the first one to question me and that he'd ask me questions like: When did I see you yesterday? Who was with Hoffman? What did you find? What does the x-ray show? I told him the x-ray didn't show much.

Then we rehearsed.

"And you saw him today?"

"Yes."

"How was he?"

"He's better but he's still sick."

"You think he could be on the stand?"

"No."

Weinglass told me that after he finished the prosecution would have at me. He added that at the end of the day, "They're going to insist on a neutral doctor to review your judgment. And you will object to whomever they put forward, and we'll have to have somebody acceptable to both sides."

People lined up around the block to see the trial. After Weinglass took me through the paces, the U.S. Attorney did have at me. He asked me if I had checked for some malady that I can't remember. I told him there was no test for that. Clever guy was trying to trip me up. As I later learned, he had several brothers who were doctors. Maybe he'd consulted with them to find out what he should ask the sly Communist.

When he was done, he went back to his table and whispered something to his aide. Davis, who had the seat closest to the prosecutors, laughed. Later he told me the guy had said, "I think he's straight." With friends like that, you don't need enemies.

In the end, just as Weinglass had predicted, the prosecution asked Judge Hoffman to allow Dr. Joseph Freilich, an expert in chest disease, to examine Abbie Hoffman. He would then provide an objective diagnosis to the court.

Weinglass started to object. He was going to argue that the doctor had to be acceptable to both sides. The defense had not been consulted about this Dr. Freilich.

I caught his attention and urged him not to object. He looked at me as if I were crazy, but he did not object.

"What's the deal?" he whispered.

I told him that Joe Freilich was an old friend and colleague. In fact, he was my doctor. Crazy, huh? But this is the story of my life, really. They take my doctor to become the expert in this criminal matter. I didn't expect Joe to do me any favors, but I expected him to be fair.

After court adjourned, we went to see the patient/defendant, who again had a companion in bed with him. Joe Freilich had already looked at the x-ray. There was a spot on Hoffman's lung that you could argue was abnormal. It wasn't necessarily something warranting hospitalization, but it was enough to create a little uncertainty.

Hoffman was holding a sputum cup.

"What's this?" Joe asked.

"Oh," Hoffman said, leering, "the girls spit in this."

Luckily Joe had a sense of humor.

Because I was a witness, I was not allowed in the courtroom to hear Freilich's testimony. But I was told he used the word "conservative" about thirty times. Bottom line: reluctant to contradict the patient's regular physician, he said that a conservative reading of the x-ray and a conservative examination of the patient could lead to the conservative, but not unreasonable, decision to hospitalize.

Phew! That may have been one of the only times somebody called me conservative, but I was glad of it. My reputation was on the line, and Judge Hoffman, whom I think even the most legitimately conservative court-watchers thought was off the curve, could have held me in contempt.

This episode begs the question: Did I behave ethically? I'd like to think I'd always draw the line between what's ethical and what's not ethical. What I was confronted with here was a patient. He was pretty sick, but not terribly so. In normal practice I would probably have told him to go home and call me and tell me how he was doing.

But this wasn't that. This was a case of being on the witness stand, which I think you can reasonable argue is an arduous, challenging thing for anybody. In my heart of hearts, I had to weigh this sick patient being on the stand, not at home resting in bed with or without other girls in the room with him. So I protected my patient. Now the patient wasn't an ordinary patient, it was Abbie Hoffman. Everything was a joke to him including my reputation as a doctor, but that didn't matter.

Another question: If the lawyers for, say, Scooter Libby had come to me and said Scooter wasn't feeling well and given me the same kind of cues that Leonard Weinglass gave me and his x-ray had looked exactly like Hoffman's, would I have come to the same conclusion?

The answer is yes. It is very important that we have a continuous, even-balanced, ethical posture.

It's also very important we have an equitable justice system. In the case of the Chicago Seven, justice was slow to come. The jury found Weiner and Froines not guilty on all charges. It found that Davis, Dellinger, Hayden, Hoffman, and Rubin had incited riots, but had not conspired to do so. Judge Hoffman weighed in, too, holding all the defendants and Kunstler and Weinglass in contempt of court and giving each of them jail time.

As the Chicago *Tribune* later reported, "Eventually all of the contempt sentences and the riot charges were either dismissed by higher courts or dropped by the government. At the time, it was the Trial of the Century, but in the end the Chicago Seven Trial seemed to mean nothing at all."

Despite going through the judicial wringer, the Chicago Seven were afforded a trial by jury. During the same month that I testified, my patient Fred Hampton, the 21-year-old deputy chairman of the Illinois chapter of the Black Panther Party, had no such opportunity.

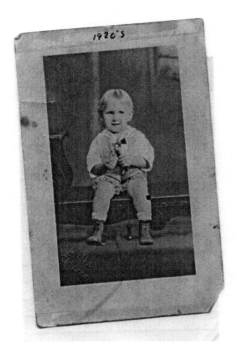

Quentin Young circa 1926

Quentin in US army, 1944

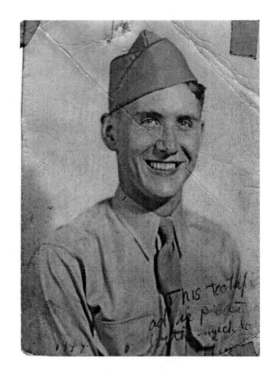

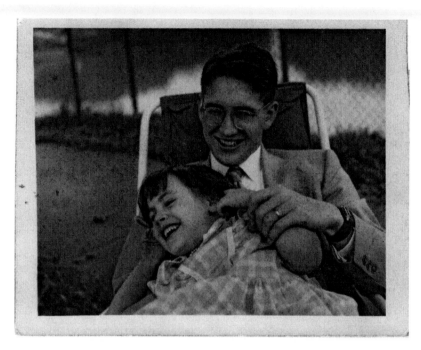

Quentin and eldest daughter Nancy, early 1950s

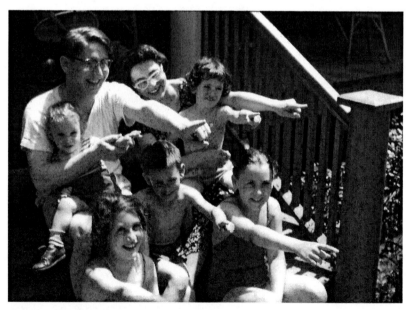

Quentin, wife Jessie and their 5 kids, 1960s

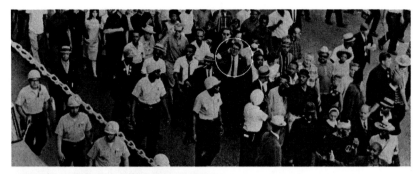

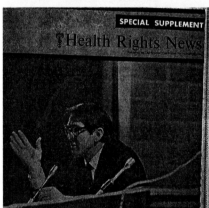

Quentin marching with Martin Luther King, Jr. in Chicago, 1965

Quentin testifying before HUAC, 1968

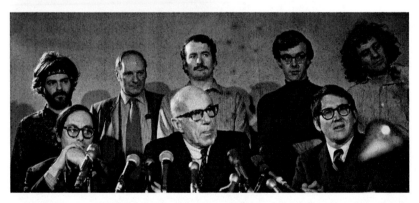

October 29, 1969 -Chicago, Illinois-Dr. Benjamin Spock (front, center), whose conviction on charges of conspiracy to commit draft evasion was recently overturned by the U.S. Court of Appeals, talks at a news conference in Chicago's Federal Building. At left is Dr. Howard Levy, recently released from prison after serving a two year sentence for refusing to train Green Beret doctors, and at right is Dr. Quentin Young from the Medical Committee for Human Rights. Standing are defendents in the Chicago Eight conspiracy trial, (left to right): Jerry Rubin, David Dellinger, John Froines, Rennie Davis and Abbie Hoffman. (Copyright Bettmann/Corbis / AP Images.)

Quentin 1970s rally in Chicago

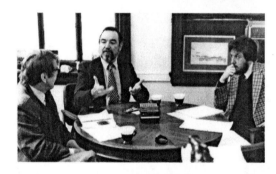

Quentin rallying support
for single-payer, 1980s
Chicago

Quentin Young, John
McKnight, Jack Salmon
-early days of HMPRG,
circa 1983

From left, John McKnight,
Studs Terkel, Pat Terrell,
and Quentin on Quentin's
public radio show, 1984

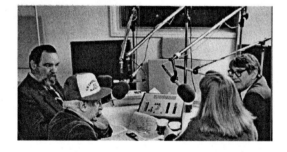

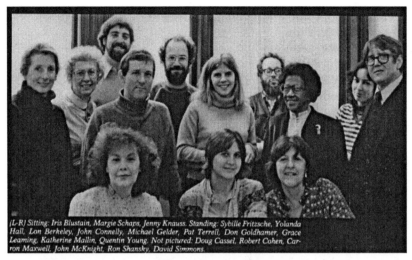

[L-R] Sitting: Iris Blustain, Margie Schaps, Jenny Knauss. Standing: Sybille Fritzsche, Yolanda Hall, Lon Berkeley, John Connelly, Michael Gelder, Pat Terrell, Don Goldhamer, Grace Leaming, Katherine Mailin, Quentin Young. Not pictured: Doug Cassel, Robert Cohen, Carron Maxwell, John McKnight, Ron Shansky, David Simmons.

Early HMPRG staff and board, 1984

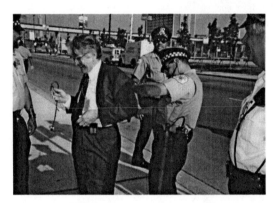

Quentin outside Democratic National Convention being frisked by police in Chicago, 1996

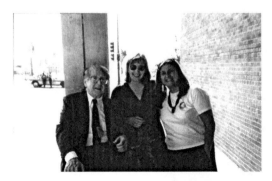

Quentin, former HMPRG executive director, Linda Diamond Shapiro, and executive director Margie Schaps outside the 1996 Democratic National Convention in Chicago

Quentin speaking outside Canadian embassy seeking medical asylum in 2004 with fellow PNHP leaders Jack Geiger and Claudia Fegan

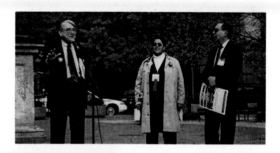

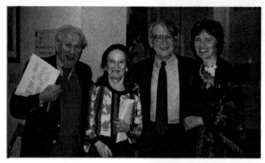

Studs Terkel and wife Ida, Quentin and Ruth, 1998 - Quentin's 75th birthday celebration

Dr. Quentin Young and PNHP Executive Director Dr. Ida Hellander at PNHP's exhibit at the American College of Physicians in 1997. Dr. Young was inducted as a "master" of the ACP that year.

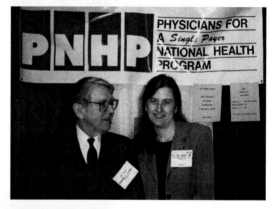

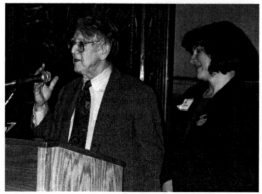

Dr. Quentin Young giving Dr. Deborah Richter from Vermont the Quentin Young health activist award at the PNHP Annual Meeting in Chicago in May 2000.

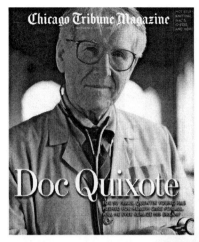

Doc Quixote Chicago *Tribune*
Magazine Cover Dec. 9, 2001

Margie Schaps, Quentin
and Studs Terkel 2003,
at HMPRG fundraiser

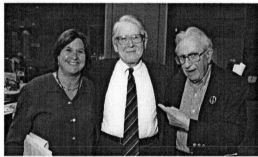

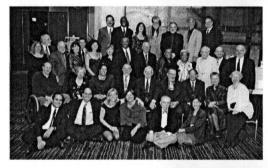

Current and former HMPRG
board 2003

Quentin and then Senate Candidate Barack Obama 2003

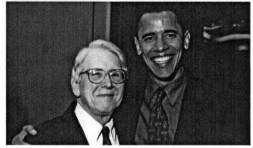

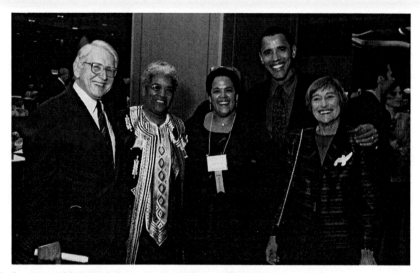

Quentin at 2003 fundraiser with Linda Murray, Claudia Fegan, IL State Senator Barack Obama and IL State Representative Barbara Flynn Currie

Quentin, with wife Ruth, sharing a laugh with Governor Pat Quinn, 2003

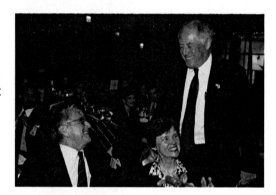

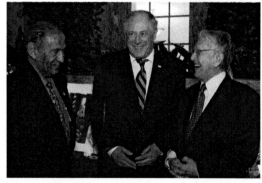

Congressman John Conyers, Governor Pat Quinn and Quentin at another fundraiser, 2005

Announcing the introduction of the "Proposal of the Physicians' Working Group for Single-Payer National Health Insurance" into Congress in the form of H.R. 676 in 2003.

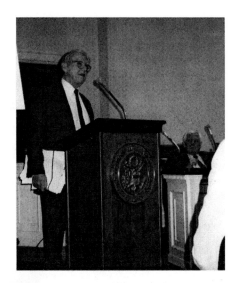

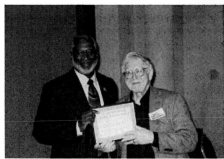

Quentin with Surgeon General Dr. David Satcher

Quentin and US Senator Barack Obama at Labor Rally March 2007, AP Image

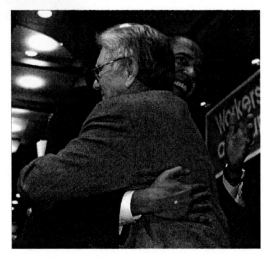

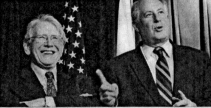

Legendary doctor retires

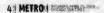

SIX-DECADE CAREER | MLK, Abbie Hoffman were patients — now health care activism is his focus

BY MIKE THOMAS
Religion Reporter/mthomas@suntimes.com

His patients have included Barack Obama, Martin Luther King and Mike Royko.

His politics are, and long have been, vocally and unabashedly liberal.

And now, after an immensely productive and sometimes tumultuous six-decade career, Dr. Quentin Young is retiring from the practice of internal medicine to focus on patient advocacy and equal health care rights — priorities he has pursued for decades.

On Friday, Illinois Lt. Gov. Pat Quinn threw a surprise news conference in Young's honor at the James R. Thompson Center, attended by 20 or so friends and colleagues.

"I have to say that despite Dr. Young's medical efforts, I'm still alive," Quinn, one of Young's patients, joked.

Formerly president of the Chicago Board of Health and Cook

County Hospital's chief medical officer, Young was fired from the latter post in the mid-'70s for siding with and speaking out on behalf of residents and interns during a 13-day strike.

He also was an ally to counterculture icons. At the end of the turbulent 1960s, Young tended to Abbie Hoffman during the renegade hippie's Chicago Seven trial and worked with the Black Panthers on a "Free Peoples' Medical Center."

In 1968, he challenged the now-infamous House Un-American Activities subcommittee to ask him whether he belonged to the Communist Party. When they did, he refused to answer. When they threatened him with contempt of

Congress, he still refused.

"My answer is that the question is an unconstitutional invasion of my rights," Young told his interrogators. "I chastise the subcommittee counsel for daring to ask the question."

Ray Wang, program director of the Chicago Area Schweitzer Fellows Program (which is associated with Young's Health and Medicine group),

called Young a "hero" and praised his profundity. "In an era when so many people are silent or sitting on their hands, he's always been vocal, but in a good way," Wang said.

Afterward, Young reminisced about his colorful career.

"The high point for me were the moments I spent with [Martin Luther] King," he said. "For reasons I can't explain, I was assigned as his doctor. That was the good news. The bad news, he never got sick very much. But the several times he had a cold, they called me and I took a 15-minute house call and made it a three-hour afternoon with the master."

Young said there was "a lot of sad business" too, including violent riots that broke out between cops during the 1968 Democratic National Convention in Chicago. "To see such a disintegration of norms was very hard."

He also spoke of his vision for the future of health care in America.

"If you look at the timeline for really big things — the end of slavery, women's suffrage, pensions, social security — they took decades. And we're closer now [to equal health care] than ever."

So he's hopeful.

"I'm more than hopeful," Young said. "I'm optimistic."

Comment at suntimes.com.

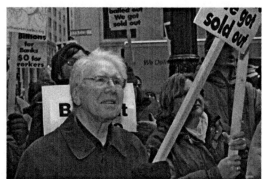
Lt. Gov. Pat Quinn (right) announces April 25 as Quentin Young Day on Friday at the Thompson Center. Young, a Hyde Park internist who is retiring, was once chief medical officer of Cook County Hospital. | JOHN J. KIM • SUN-TIMES

Chicago Sun-Times Clipping 2008 Quentin and Governor Pat Quinn upon Quentin's retirement

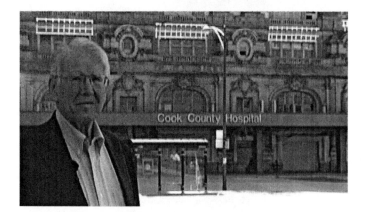

Quentin and Margie Schaps supporting Republic Windows Workers, 2008

Quentin 2009 in front of the old Cook County Hospital

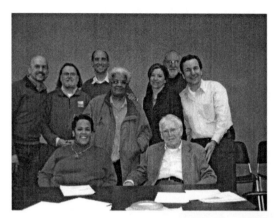

HMPRG Executive
Committee 2011

Richard Sewell, Quentin
Young, Linda Murray, US
Representative Jan
Schakowsky 2011

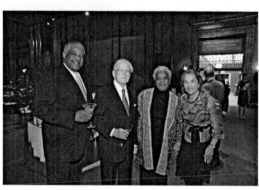

Eight

If he had lived, would Fred Hampton have become another Martin Luther King? The second coming of Malcolm X? We'll never know. A little before 5 a.m. on December 4, 1969, Fred and fellow Panther Mark Clark died during a police raid masterminded by Cook County State's Attorney Edward Hanrahan. According to witnesses, Fred had been slipped barbiturates by an FBI mole and was asleep when a team of fourteen cops burst through the doors of his West Side apartment. Wounded in the initial hail of bullets, he was dragged from his bedroom and shot to death, said another Black Panther who was in the apartment.

Prior to the tragedy, the FBI had given the State's Attorney a blueprint of Hampton's apartment. Hanrahan himself was later indicted on charges related to the raid—obstructing justice and conspiracy to present false evidence. And thirteen years after the murders, a jury in a civil suit found that the government conspired to deprive Fred and other victims of the raid of their civil rights. The jury awarded $2 million to the survivors and the families of Hampton and Clark.

Thanks to my work with MCHR, I had the privilege of getting to know many of the leaders of the civil rights movement from Martin Luther King, Jr. to Fannie Lou Hamer to Stokely Carmichael. It may come as a surprise when I say that Fred Hampton was as charismatic as any of these luminaries. I don't want to romanticize him, but he was a great communicator possessed of an almost unequaled combination of intelligence, street smarts, political savvy, youthful vigor, charm, and leadership skills.

To be sure, Fred was a member of the Black Panther Party (BPP), a group that most people associated with incendiary language and stockpiles of weapons. But if you listened closely to what Fred was saying, you heard the most extraordinary message. At a time when much of the African American community was going beyond black pride and black unity to a movement for black separatism, Fred emphatically appealed for white participation and support in the numerous projects that he and his colleagues were putting together.

This was counter-current. Visionary. He was asking all people to participate in the effort to organize and elevate the most downtrodden sectors of our society. That certainly appealed to me.

Fred and I met when the paths of MCHR and the BPP merged in an effort to achieve a common goal: delivering health care to the most disadvantaged among us. In the late 1960s, our Committee and their party were committed to opening free clinics in needy neighborhoods across the country. In fact, we'd been at it for a year or two by the time the Panthers approached us. So, too, had other MCHR chapters and local groups across the country.

People's (or community) clinics were based on indigenous activity. Thanks to other initiatives like the free breakfast program, the Panthers were skilled at engaging their constituency. As a result the BPP had a rather clear notion of what it wanted: a free clinic in the community where its largest number of supporters and members were, a clinic where people could come for care in a way that they couldn't get elsewhere.

My initial contact was not Fred, but a most un-Panther-like Panther named Ronald "Doc" Satchel. Doc, who eventually became the Chicago chapter's "Minister of Health," was still a teenager, modest, unassuming, soft spoken, and slight. He stood 5'6" or 5'7" tall and weighed 120 pounds dripping wet. (That body would end up wounded in the raid that killed Fred.)

Al Raby, the ex-teacher who had become the leader of CCCO, sent Doc to me. Al told me to expect a young black student interested in health issues. And that's what I got. Doc didn't yet have a lot of formal knowledge on the subject, but he had a commitment to launching clinics in the community following the model of the breakfast programs and clinics that the party had recently opened in California. He wanted to know how to go about doing it in

Chicago and to learn everything about the free clinic movement.

We talked and then I gave him some books, telling him what I tell everybody I lend books to: "The only way to really make me dislike you is to fail to return your books. If you return them, I'll give you more." He returned them. I gave him more.

Not too long after meeting with Doc, I met Fred and some of the other leaders of the Chicago chapter. Fred was an item on the West Side. He was active in the NAACP youth. When the Panthers came along, he gravitated towards their more militant doctrine.

First time I saw him was at a church on Ashland Avenue where he was giving a lecture. His charisma was immediately apparent. He delivered his message differently than many traditional leaders, moving about the stage with great energy, bringing the audience with him as he talked about racism and the desire to have a more equitable world.

The Panthers had an office at MCHR headquarters where Fred began working with Doc to develop a clinic. We talked about the particulars of such an undertaking and the details of the physical plant: What the space would look like. The need for something attractive. Nothing that looked jerry-built. No rundown equipment. Brick-layering to replace the storefront wall.

About a year after I first met Fred, he was busted for distributing allegedly stolen ice cream bars to kids in the neighborhood. He went to jail. After his release, he was brought to me for a physical evaluation. He charmed everyone in our office.

After Fred was murdered, there was a big outpouring of support that facilitated the construction of the clinic on the West Side. My role? Using my contacts to find recruits and in-kind support—whether it was volunteering professional time or liberating, in the best sense, equipment, supplies, drugs, and medicines.

I loved the idea of the clinic, was impressed that people were fashioning their own solutions to their own problems. The Panthers weren't taking the easy route. The community they picked, Lawndale, was about as depressed as you can get in America. It was the center of the ghetto. Very high joblessness, a very high dependency on welfare, all of the attendant problems.

Many Chicagoans, black and white, thought the Panthers too militant, but we had no trouble attracting people to serve in the clinic. The Panthers had an extraordinary appeal to many young doctors who were either in training at the hospitals or already out in practice, as well as nurses, technicians, and all the elements that go into a well-run medical center. The patients certainly were willing to come.

Debbie Wei of civilrightsteaching.org has assembled old BPP handouts that detail the history and programs of the Party. The following handout, titled "People's Medical Care Center," was written by Lincoln Webster Sheffield and appeared in *The Black Panther* on October 26, 1968. It presents an excellent snapshot of the clinic.

"One of the Black Panther Party programs in Chicago is the People's Medical Care Center, located in the Lawndale ghetto on the West Side. The center is named for Spurgeon 'Jake' Winters, a martyred Panther killed by police last year.

The only publicity the center has received came when city authorities attempted to close it a few days after it opened in December, charging numerous building and Board of Health violations. But the center remains open, in spite of harassment, and it regularly treats more than 100 patients every week.

Part of the center's work includes training community people to perform services wherever possible. 'For example,' said Mrs. Woods, one of the center's volunteers, 'we are training some of the young people to do laboratory urinalysis and blood tests, and teams of people from the community are organized to canvass the neighborhood and bring the center to the people. Most of the people in Lawndale are so poor they never go to a doctor until they are practically dying. Our teams take their blood pressure, medical histories, and in general determine if there are people suffering from illness. If illness is discovered, whether chronic or just simple ailments, the person is urged to visit the center, where an examination, treatment, and prescription are all free.'

In a typical evening of duty, Mrs. Woods may help to treat 20 or 30 people. One patient, she said, brought in a four-month old baby who had a bad cold. The baby was examined by the pediatrician, and a throat culture was taken. This baby had been going to the well-baby clinic operated by the Board of Health, but had not yet received any of the normal shots. After the examination and discussion with the mother, an appointment was made for the baby to return for continued treatment and shots. Mrs. Woods said all of the patients were treated free, no questions asked about 'ability to pay' or anything. On hand to take care of all these people were a pediatrician, a general practitioner, two interns, and two nurses.

The center does not stop at treating medical problems. A member of the Black Panther Party is on hand at all times to serve as a 'people's advocate.' He interviews each patient.

'Whenever possible, the Panthers will help with the problem, no matter what it is,' Mrs. Woods said. 'For example, we discovered that many of the school children, aside from problems like going without breakfast, faced serious strain from the difficulty of finding a place to study or play, safe from the hazards of the street. So we opened up the center to them during the afternoon, before the regular hours, where they can play quietly, or study, paint or do whatever they wish.'

The success of the Spurgeon 'Jake' Winters People's Medical Care Center has inspired similar efforts by other organizations, particularly those in the 'rainbow coalition' with the Panthers. Both the Young Lords and the Young Patriots have opened centers, although they are not yet operating as full a schedule as the Panthers."

I came to the clinic weekly. By every standard, I was a senior citizen—in my mid-forties. Believe it or not, having been in practice perhaps some twenty years, I was by way of presentation, and by way of conducting myself professionally, very much a conservative—wearing a three-piece suit without, I hope, being particularly haughty. I just felt that was the way I'd like to do it.

Most of the other doctors and volunteer staff thought and dressed differently. Blue jeans were the norm. Shirts could be clean, but never pressed. Ties were a sign of selling out. Wearing sandals or even going barefoot was okay.

Make no mistake, these young lions and lionesses were dedicated and skilled. They simply liked this idea of organic unity with the patients. But let the record show that these patients, for all their poverty, were neater, dressed better, and were more concerned about their presentation than the doctors.

I relate this to make a point. Doc Satchel ran the clinic. About two weeks after the opening, Doc called all the doctors into the break area and said he wanted to tell us something. We expected a pronouncement of import, perhaps some major change in policy. I can't remember the exact words he used, but he said something like this: "I got a problem. We have a lot of patients who come here that see doctors. They see them in the clinics, they see them in their doctor's office on occasion, and those doctors present themselves with white coats, stethoscopes and even ties. And you're confusing these patients. So, what we've done is get a large assortment of doctor jackets for you."

Doc pointed to a rack that had at least fifty jackets of all sizes and colors. "Pick the one you like, but we'll expect you to wear a jacket here so the patients will understand that by the outward symbols you are indeed a doctor in addition to your great desire to serve the people." Serve the people was, of course, a Panther slogan. Young Doc was not being sarcastic, but ironic.

There was some grumbling from the professional volunteers about being too bourgeois and selling out, but they got the point and started wearing the jackets. And while it's a small point, it does remind us that if you're going to serve the people, don't give them added burdens of worrying about whether you're a real doctor because you don't dress like any doctor they ever saw. It's an indulgence on your part to demand that they accept you as you try and mimic what you think their style is.

I like to think that our clinic in Lawndale helped inspire the BPP to "go national." In her book, *Body and Soul: The Black Panther Party and the Fight Against Medical Discrimination,* Professor Alondra Nelson writes:

"By 1970, People's Free Medical Clinics had become a requirement for every BPP chapter. In 1972, the BPP revised point six of the founding 10 point platform, adding a demand for: completely free health care for all black and oppressed people...We believe that the government must provide, free of charge, for the people, health facilities which will not only treat our illnesses, most of which have come about as a result of our oppression, but which will also develop preventative medical programs to guarantee our future survival. We believe that mass health education and research programs must be developed to give black and oppressed people access to advanced scientific and medical information, so we may provide ourselves with proper medical attention and care."

Sadly Fred did not live to see this. As I told the press years ago, "This is a terrible way to put it, but the people who made it their business to kill the leaders of the black movement picked the right ones."

Before his death, Fred was responsible for inspiring another group of urban activists to open clinics in Chicago's Lincoln Park area. Originally a gang, the Young Lords had evolved into a party pushing for Puerto Rican independence and a better way of life for Puerto Ricans in the mainland United States. Along with the Young Patriots (which represented poor whites in Chicago), the Lords joined a Rainbow Coalition created by Fred and the Panthers. (This is not to be confused with the Rainbow Coalition formed by the Reverend Jesse Jackson some years later.)

Along with Dr. Jack Johns, Ana Lucas, and Alberto and Marta Chavarria, I helped the Young Lords open a free health clinic in February of 1970. MCHR again helped staff the operation.

In his article, "From Gang-bangers to Urban Revolutionaries: The Young Lords of Chicago," Judson Jeffries describes the effort:

"The clinic served nearly fifty people every Saturday, with services from prenatal care to eye examinations. At first some residents were reluctant to visit the clinic. They were still leery of the Lords' old gang image and were frightened by what they read in the newspapers.

Recognizing their credibility problem, the Young Lords started canvassing door-to-door, asking residents if anyone needed medical care and making arrangements for them to go to the clinic. If the people failed to appear, they were sent a follow-up letter inviting them to visit the clinic. Some of the time, members of the Health Ministry and doctors would make house calls, especially for those whose mobility was restricted.

Initially Grant Hospital (an area hospital) agreed to provide free follow-up examinations upon referral by the clinic's doctors. But the hospital soon began billing the clinic patients and initiating collection procedures. Consequently, the Lords severed its relationship with the hospital. By that time, however, the Lords had earned the trust of the people and were able to increase the level of its services in order to meet the community's growing needs. Through the Health Clinic the Lords were able to strengthen their bond with the community and to expose the inadequacies of the established social service institutions."

As evidenced by the Panther and Young Lords clinics, there were a lot of young health care students and professionals (and more than a few old geezers like myself) dedicated to improving the delivery of services to underserved communities and eliminating the inequality of service based on race, socioeconomic status, and gender. A thought occurred: Could we marry the medical curriculum with social and political questions? And so, with the help of a grant from the Carnegie Corporation of New York, was born the Urban Preceptorship Program (UPP) at the University of Illinois-Chicago, where I was on the faculty.

Here's an excerpt from a 1970 article I wrote for *The New Physician* describing the program:

"It is a painful truth that health science students in general and medical students in particular complete all of their undergraduate, graduate, and postgraduate education to levels of exquisite specialization only to enter a complex, crisis-ridden system of health care with the naivete of a newborn....

Reasoning that the special problems of health care to the

excluded community—the poor, the black, the aged—might be alleviated by analyzing and mastering the urban arrangements for delivery of health care, (we) have devised a course for senior health science students (mainly medical students) from all over the country. Called the Urban Preceptorship Program, this course harkens back to an ancient and sometimes discredited mode of instruction, the preceptorship. While spurning the live-in apprentice quality characterizing the outlawed preceptorship of (earlier) times, the positive aspects of the preceptorship—intimacy, collegiality, accessibility—are sought."

I went on to describe a three-month course that was to be taught four times a year. Relying heavily on the seminar technique, it began with three weeks "consumed by day-long, intense rap sessions with an array of health care savants" ranging from the commissioner of health of Chicago to a board member of a local center to a pediatrician practicing in the ghetto. Students then had the freedom to pick an area for ten weeks of field work.

The choices were, I wrote, "excitingly varied." One student analyzed the power structure at Cook County Hospital. Another evaluated the relationships of the "spate of free health clinics in the city to major institutions, proposing a contractual arrangement covering clinic funding and patient referral." A third student developed a "thoughtful proposal for community nominations for medical school admissions in the Chicago area."

I concluded that the response to the program during its first year had been "unexpectedly strong." It had already grown from four students per quarter to eleven, and we planned to enlarge the number to 24 the following year.

UPP was a great success. We received a large grant from the Nixon administration, and we expanded the scope of the course work to include courses on "Health Care in the Urban Setting," "Legal Foundations of Public Health and Medical Care," and "Prison Medicine." As hoped, UPP spawned independent community health organizations. Several women in the project joined Chicago Women's Liberation Union, an organization focused on women's health and reproductive rights. And after the Supreme

Court's 1973 decision in *Roe v. Wade,* women from the UPP created HERS (Health Evaluation and Referral Service) to help women find safe abortion clinics.

Federal funding for the program waned as the country trended to the right. Today, the Schweitzer Fellows Program at HM-PRG draws on many of the principles of the UPP. More about this later.

I hope I've conveyed the fact that in the 1960s there was a real movement to improve the health care of the disadvantaged. A couple of other examples: at the same time the Panthers were opening clinics, The National Health Council held its annual forum. The forum always focused on a "select national health problem," and in 1969 the topic was "Health Problems of the Inner City." Representatives from the community, the medical world, government, academia, the private sector, and the union movement met in New York.

The purpose? "The Council is aware that the President's Commission on Civil Disorders did not emphasize the role of health services in the problems which the United States now faces in the urban slums. Numerous conferences, new organizations, and new programs are testimony to the significance of these problems and reinforce the Council's belief that the problem is far from solution and urgent as a national priority."

The focus? "A realistic assessment of the challenge which the inner city presents to our present health care industry, including: experiments in organizing and delivering of services such as neighborhood health centers…. The Forum is planned to stimulate action as a result of deliberation."

And the program? "(An) opportunity for pooling and exchange of information on the nature and dimension of health problems that have been defined by inner city residents and health care professionals concerned with these problems."

I was one of those many concerned professionals. That year I served on the Forum planning committee. I also met with groups of the inner city residents in Chicago before and after the conference. Everybody kept saying they wanted services, clinics and cost controls. We tried to deliver.

Another initiative: At the same time that UPP was getting its legs, MCHR was starting to focus on the human rights of prisoners. This went beyond making sure that the incarcerated received basic medical treatment. Our organization was responding to the California Department of Corrections' consideration of employing "some of the more exotic branches of anatomy and the social sciences" to address the very real problem of violence within the prison. To our dismay, the chief of the Department's Research Division wanted to discuss "research into the etiology of violent behavior and how corrective measures can be developed to modify the condition... such things as organic brain dysfunction... visually evoked potential, pathological intoxication, disturbances of stress tolerance, behavior modification efforts, anthropological studies all might come into consideration."

If you are having a hard time wrapping your head around this, I have six words for you: *One Flew Over the Cuckoo's Nest*. Our point here was that "the cure has become the cancer." For these and other efforts, MCHR was under FBI surveillance for years. I have the files!

As involved as I was with MCHR, the clinics, and the UPP, I continued my private practice in Hyde Park. After doing my rounds early in the morning at Michael Reese, I would return to Hyde Park and see patients. My office in the Hyde Park Bank building was like the offices of most of my internal medicine peers, predictable. There was a receptionist desk, a waiting room, a couple of examining rooms, posters of Lenin and Trotsky. I joke. There were no such posters on the wall, only my diplomas.

I was never at a loss for patients. I'll leave it to others to speculate as to whether that was because there was a doctor's shortage or because, for better or worse, I had a higher public profile than others or because I had a lot of social and political friends and was fortunate that patients referred family and friends. I certainly never participated in causes or protested vocally in an effort to drum up business. On the contrary, I suspect there may have been some folks who decided not to see me professionally because of my political stands.

Like Hyde Park, my practice was socioeconomically and racially diverse. Perhaps 30 to 40 percent of my patients were black. This was never an issue with the powers that be at Michael Reese. Though known as the Jewish hospital in the 1950s and '60s, Reese was located on the edge of a large African American population center and counted many blacks among its patients. (However, years later when Reese's Jewish patient base vanished, the hospital saw hard times. It was sold and re-sold, eventually to mega-health concern Humana with disastrous results. Today the hospital is no more and the land is vacant. More on this later.)

My joy and comfort and satisfaction mostly lay in seeing all kinds of people with all kinds of illnesses. Hyde Park offered me diversity of patients in urban Chicago. If you are downtown, you tend to be a monotone kind of doctor with a monotone patient load. A mingled practice is uncommon except in a place like Hyde Park, where you'll see a professor who is a head of a department, and then a working guy, and then a welfare mother. I also had adolescents, whom I really enjoyed.

It became clear to me that there was no age group I liked best, no gender I preferred (at least medically), and no disease entities that I thought, "Gee, this is for me." In a word, I gloried in "generalism."

I always saw County Hospital as a mother with open arms to any child—wounded, sick, infirm. No barrier—economic or otherwise. There may be the barrier of a six-hour wait, which is a barrier to be sure, but you never have the option of saying, "My schedule is full," or "I don't see these kind of patients," or "I don't take blacks." As a primary care doctor in private practice, I tried to adopt that same approach.

As I was settling into my practice, the trend towards specialization was gaining momentum. The specialists were earning more money than we generalists. This inequity created a modest kind of class-consciousness, a built-in hierarchy of economic inequality. By and large the generalists worked harder, longer hours and had more demands from patients than did the typical specialist. Maybe this should have bothered me or made me jealous, but I was quite content.

Why? It struck me that most of the people who did the sub-specialized stuff had a very limited world view as far as medical gratification, a world that to me seemed tedious and narrow. Don't get me wrong, I don't mean to dismiss the excitement of fixing say a crippled hip into a fully usable limb, but I've never been able to understand, no matter how great the economic reward, how an otherwise normal human being could do that all day, every day. (Lest you think these are the musings of a cranky old man, I must note that I expressed these in an interview with my friend and colleague Fitzhugh Mullan many moons ago.)

And while I am taking a few shots at my brothers and sisters who are surgeons, here's another one: they're dealing with their patients when they are asleep! That doesn't seem to me a particularly attractive side of medical practice.

I was fortunate to be a kind of Zelig to a number of accomplished and well-known Chicagoans and outsiders. Locally, I counted author/raconteur Studs Terkel and columnist Mike Royko among my patients. Seeing these people in the examining room was an enormous opportunity. While Royko never tired of mocking my radical ideas, we got along very well as doctor, patient, and friends. This was true with Studs as well, who was full of stories. He kept going into his nineties. He was much more congenial to my particular ideas. (I also ministered to the Beatles when they were performing in town. A Chicago producer, Frank Fried, invited me to be their physician. This was most interesting to my kids, who wanted to go to their shows.)

While tuberculosis was the scourge in my medical school and County years, polio was the killer during my early years of practice. In 1952, there were some 58,000 cases. More than 3,100 people died from the disease and another 20,000 were left with some form of paralysis. One thing about polio: it didn't respect a person's class or standing in the community. People who would be immune to most of the socially caused diseases weren't immune to polio. Case in point: my med school classmate, County roommate, Tom Sheridan got polio. Fortunately, he recovered.

Polio wasn't something you read about that was afflicting people in Africa or downstate Illinois, it was epidemic in Chicago.

Combine that with the fact that the disease often left its mark on its victims for life and you have a phenomenon that got everybody's attention.

I have always been a strong believer in preventive medicine. But until a vaccine was developed, prevention was impossible. You could only treat polio after it presented itself.

And then... In April of 1955, those monitoring trials of a vaccine developed by Dr. Jonas Salk pronounced the vaccine "safe and effective." In the pre-Internet, pre-24/7 cable news world, news spread fast. Church bells rang. Workplaces observed moments of silence. The pharmaceutical giant Eli Lilly even paid a quarter of a million dollars to broadcast the news via closed circuit to over 50,000 doctors gathered in movie theatres across the country.

The Polio Fund, which many people know as the March of Dimes, had previously announced it would purchase nine million doses of the vaccine for the free immunization of children and pregnant women. There was one contingency: doctors could not charge a fee for administering the vaccine. Believe it or not, some medical societies initially balked at the no fee stipulation.

Some in the medical establishment debated whether mass inoculations were necessary. They pointed to declining incidence of polio. In Chicago, Health Commissioner Bundeson took the opposite position. He asked anybody who knew how to administer a vaccine by injection to volunteer. And of course many nurses and many doctors like myself did respond.

By July of 1969, I was so fed up with the AMA that I told the New York *Times*, "I've been an AMA member since 1959 and I just can't justify my membership any longer. I had been one of those who tried to work for reform inside the structure, but we just couldn't do it. They (AMA leaders) are captives of the right wing. The organization is exceedingly undemocratic."

The occasion of the article, which ran under the headline, "Protester likens AMA to Saigon Government," was the organization's annual convention. Other doctors "contended that association policy had thwarted free inoculations to the poor, disregarded programs designed to aid the poor, and perpetuated the conception of 'illness as a marketable commodity.'"

A word about preventive medicine in general. In the mid-20th century, doctors focused their attention on treating the illnesses that patients presented. The prevention movement, while respected, was in its early stages. You didn't hear of too many doctors warning their patients about the risks of obesity, for example. There was little screening of random populations for high cholesterol, diabetes, or hypertension.

And what about smoking? Surf the Internet and you will find that from the 1920s to the 1950s, many publications, including the *Journal of the American Medical Association,* featured advertisements in which doctors extolled cigarettes. Just one example: A doctor in lab coat, cigarette in hand, looking very contented next to the headline: "More Doctors Smoke Camels than any Other Cigarette." The *JAMA* finally stopped taking such ads in 1953. This was just about the time that early studies were beginning to show the health risks of smoking and suggesting a link to lung cancer.

I'm happy to report that I was able to quit in 1955 at age 32 after smoking for half my life. And when I did quit I became a zealot, preaching to my patients to stop.

It's one thing to be able to influence the few hundred patients that might be in your practice. It's quite another to impact thousands on a daily basis, especially if those thousands don't have access to private physicians. I didn't go looking for the opportunity to have this greater impact. But when it presented itself in a most improbable way, I took the chance.

Nine

On April 1, 1969, the following headline appeared in the Chicago *Tribune*: COOK COUNTY HOSPITAL REFORM BILL SENT TO OGILVIE. Sounds like a cruel April Fools Day joke, doesn't it? The hospital, in a state of disrepair and despair, facing an increasingly angry and vocal staff and community, certainly was in need of the state's intervention. But who could believe that the Democratic Machine that controlled the institution's lucrative purse strings and patronage rolls would allow their minions in the state legislature to support the newly-elected Republican Governor Richard Ogilvie's reform plan?

Yet it was no hoax. The times they were a changin' at County. And soon, I'd be part of that change.

Ogilvie was no stranger to the machinations at the hospital. In 1966, while serving as sheriff of Cook County, he successfully ran for County board president. And when he ran for governor two years later, he made depoliticizing the hospital a cornerstone of his candidacy. Thanks in large part to the testimony of County's house staff (interns and residents), legislators could no longer ignore the need to put management of the hospital into the hands of managers instead of politicians.

At the time, no one wanted the place to go under. If County sank, where would its patients go? To the private hospitals across the city? Heaven forbid.

The County Hospitals Governing Commission Act of 1969 transferred control of the hospital, as well as Oak Forest Hospital, Cermak Hospital and the Cook County Department of Corrections, to the Health and Hospitals Governing Commission

(HHGC). A nine-member independent commission that included the deans of Chicago area medical schools? That was the good news. The bad news was that the County Board rather than the HHGC retained control of the budget and personnel.

In 1971, the Board hired 45 year-old Dr. James Haughton as Executive Director of HHGC. He was responsible to the governing commission, but word was he had carte blanche to fix what all acknowledged was a floundering institution. (As the Chicago *Sun-Times* would later report, many of his meetings with the commission lasted less than twenty minutes. There was no question about who was in charge.)

Jim Haughton had previously been first deputy administrator of the New York Health and Welfare Department. In the years that followed, we worked together and we clashed. We were, I guess, friendly enemies. I've never read a better description of him than the one written by Judith Barnard in a 1976 piece for *Chicago* magazine:

"James Haughton cultivates a mercurial personality as assiduously as a boxer works on technique. He switches rapidly from charming openness with wide, if not innocent, eyes to barely controlled anger; from quiet, head-tipping listening to a stream of non-substantive phrases elegantly expressed; from insouciance to a flood of tears. Tall, imposing, with the build of an athlete, the hands of a musician, and white mutton-chop sideburns etched against polished brown skin, he dresses in leather suits of gleaming black or ivory or silver or green, matching suede shirts or turtleneck sweaters or exotically flowered shirts open to—as one doctor put it—his umbilicus...."

That was Jim, all right. To which I would add: he understood the political side of big medicine, but he was too often capricious. And, in my humble opinion, he was not as dedicated to the doctors and patients in his control as he should have been.

Jim's capriciousness was evident from the start of his tenure, several months before I came on board. His plan, as reported in the newspapers, was to downsize County into a 500-bed hospital with most of the care provided by a full-time staff. This new community hospital would "have links to neighborhood health centers." In essence this would eliminate most of the house staff and end County's long-time role/mission as a teaching hospital, where as the *Tribune* noted, "students are trained to be doctors and care is provided to the multitudes who come to its doors."

Jim may have had what he thought was the best interest of the hospital in mind or he may have been trying to show that it was the administration, not the doctors, that was in charge of the hospital. Maybe both. Whatever his motive, the announcement triggered protest from the full-time staff (attendings and department chairs) as well as the house staff.

The fall of 1971 was a disaster for the hospital. In mid-October, my old med school classmate Rolf Gunnar officially "resigned" as chair of the Department of Medicine. I may not have agreed with Rolf's politics, but I had great respect for his skill as a cardiologist and as the leader of one of County's most important departments.

The Department of Medicine boasted the most beds (450) in the hospital and oversaw internal medicine as well as all the internal medicine-related departments. County gave a huge amount of responsibility to the chair of the department, including overseeing the business side and recruiting the house staff. Each year we took in seventy interns. The department included more than 200 house staff in the medical residency program, fellows in dermatology, endocrinology, gastroenterology/hepatology, urology, cardiology, neurology, nephrology, etc., and the general attendings and specialists who supervised them.

"Ousted" is a better word to describe Rolf Gunnar's departure than "resigned." He had been at odds with the new administration from the beginning, stating publicly that he was alarmed by Haughton's policy decisions and imperious way of doing business. Arguing that County's viability, as well as success, was contingent on its ability to attract a strong house staff, Rolf told the *Tribune*, "If something dramatic isn't done to change the administrative structure of this hospital so that doctors have confidence in it again and can see a long-term future, then I think it will close."

He even called for Haughton's resignation.

Haughton responded with the charge that Rolf and other doctors were engaged in "guerilla warfare... using the patients as pawns of medical power politics." On November 1, he fired five of those "guerillas": staff doctors Chris Casten, Sherwood Gorbach, and Hal Levine and house doctors Bill Towne and Nick Rango, officers of the Residents and Interns Association. All were part of Rolf's department, where Haughton alleged that staff was allowing the hospital to become overcrowded as a form of protest. The quintet went to court to get their jobs back, and 300 doctors threatened to resign if their colleagues weren't reinstated.

I watched all this tumult from afar. As someone who cherished County—despite all its problems—I was troubled by Rolf's ouster, the firings, and the threats of mass resignations. I'd been pleased to see the establishment of the HHGC, but I feared that Haughton might not be the guy to turn the hospital around. The thought of returning to County on a full-time basis, with Haughton as my boss, never entered my mind. I had enough on my plate with my own practice, launching the Urban Preceptorship Program, and presiding nationally over MCHR activities, which included lobbying for an end to the war in Vietnam.

Little did I know that a conspiracy was afoot. Unbeknownst to me, Rango, who retained his position at the hospital pending the decision of a special hearing commission, approached Haughton and told him in so many words: *The only way for you to save your own ass is to appoint Quentin Young as chairman of the Department of Medicine.* According to Nick, Haughton responded by saying something to the effect, *Isn't he a communist?* (Nick passed away in 1993 at the age of 49 after a distinguished career as the director of New York State's AIDS program.)

More accurately, I was a country doctor active in organizing people in health care for the poor—which is almost as negative a credential as being a communist when it comes to being appointed chair of medicine at County. But Nick convinced Haughton that the best way to stem the flow of doctor departures and to attract terrific new doctors committed to the community was to hire me.

As part of his strategy to reform County, Nick made an analogous argument to me. I was the guy to save County, he insisted. He appealed to my politically concerned side: *This is your chance to serve the people and help young doctors have an orientation towards serving the poor.* Flattering. But I wasn't certain of that, and I saw more red flags than green ones.

First off, I didn't want to be a traitor to Rolf by taking a post from which he had been unfairly forced out. A conversation with Rolf, however, eliminated that concern. He wasn't enthusiastic about the future of County, but he made it clear that he did not see me as a Benedict Arnold.

(Sadly, one close friend did view me as a turncoat and our relationship crumbled. Hal Levine was a pulmonologist who had been at County for all the dark days preceding the governing commission. He was justifiably angered and devastated by Rolf's departure and, to my chagrin, by my acceptance of the post. In his eyes, I had crossed the picket line of those striking out against Haughton to become a card-carrying member of the establishment, part of the despised Haughton's team. Committed to County, Hal remained at the hospital after Rolf's departure—one of the few really good staff doctors who did. A few years later, when he announced he was leaving, I pleaded with him to stay and offered him the chairmanship of pulmonary medicine. I had great regard for his talent and his programmatic commitment. But he had never forgiven me for accepting the medical department chairmanship, and he left to join Rolf at Loyola. He died shortly after that in 1976 at the age of 46.)

Nick Rango was an operator—and I mean that in the most positive way. He enlisted my girlfriend of the time (I'd been divorced for about ten years) and they both started working on me to take the job. They managed to break down my common sense and persuade me to consider the post.

Of course, I consulted with others, principally the people in the Committee to End Discrimination in Chicago's Medical Institutions (CEDCMI). CEDCMI was still active. We were, in fact, the most important lay group lobbying to keep County open and get adequate funding.

The idea that I might go to County tantalized the progressive health movement. By and large, with the exception of Levine, my fellow activists were in favor of the move. Nobody else said, "Don't do it, it's a death trap," or "You don't want to go and become part of the establishment." A variety of arguments that might have been raised did not get raised.

And so I went to meet Jim Haughton in his palatial office at County. At this first encounter I found him to be a genial guy—in contrast to the legendary Karl Meyer, who had a mean streak and temper. Jim was also forthright, exhibiting no remorse whatsoever for having forced Rolf Gunnar's resignation.

When interviewing for a job in the lion's den, it's best to make all your demands upfront; in all likelihood you're never going to get another chance to lobby for the staff and prerogatives that you want. I made it clear to Jim that my number one priority was for the hospital to establish health care clinics in the neighborhoods.

In 1971, County had no such clinics. Its sole outpatient facility, the behemoth Fantus Clinic, sat on its grounds. That's where people from across the city came for post-surgery or post-hospitalization follow-up visits or were referred to from the ER. There was nothing wrong with Fantus, but, mind you, the County of Cook encompasses a huge geographic area. It was essential that we move from the one campus County Hospital environment to satellites that were nearer to our population.

Haughton agreed to meet this demand. (And he kept his promise. When I left County some ten years later, we had four neighborhood clinics. They were independent and comprehensive—far more than just a doctor and a desk. The effort continued after I left under the leadership of the talented hospital CEO Ruth Rothstein.)

Staffing was another issue we addressed at that first meeting. The hospital had a big personnel problem; in the wake of Rolf's departure and the firings, doctors were leaving in large numbers. And with the direction, if not the existence, of the hospital in limbo, few young doctors were knocking down the doors for internships or residencies.

As chief of medicine, I would have to recruit a house staff

that was large enough and talented enough to serve our patients. I'd also have to find (or retain) attendings and chiefs of various specialties like cardiology, gastroenterology, neurology, and dermatology. Rango and others had convinced Haughton that I was the magnet to attract these folks.

I was, in retrospect, overly optimistic that I could quickly recruit an A-Team of physicians. My confidence did not spring from a belief that there was a legion of doctors chomping at the bit to work for me. Rather, after eight years of involvement with MCHR (of which I was currently national president), I knew there was a large corps of physicians across the country committed to civil rights and the expansion of health services to the poor. Surely, I told myself, many of these would want to sign on for the coming adventure at County.

With Jim Haughton willing to meet my upfront demands and with the encouragement of the progressive community, I didn't really have a reason to say no. Salary would not be an issue. Nor would the complications of closing down my practice.

My salary was to be $45,000 a year. That doesn't sound like a lot today. It's my understanding that department chairs at County circa the 21st century make $300,000 or $400,000 a year. Whether it was my left-wing ideology or my eternal optimism, I was not going to haggle over my proposed paycheck. I hadn't entered medicine to make a killing, just to earn a comfortable living and, I hoped, do some good.

Leaving the practice was not a problem, either. By this time I was in a group with several other internists. They were excellent doctors, and I felt comfortable leaving my patients in their hands. My partners were supportive of my proposed move. We looked upon it as more leave of absence than resignation.

Of course, as noted in Chapter One, I almost didn't make it to County. The deed seemed to be done. Haughton had made me an offer, and I had accepted it. But as I was getting ready to go out of town, my boss-to-be said that some of the members of the governing commission would like to meet me before I assumed the new position. It wasn't a big deal, he assured me, just a get-to-know-you session.

It became a big deal when I told them I was going to North Vietnam.

I explained that this was an MCHR trip. We wanted to have a friendship with the Vietnamese people rather than bomb them, so we would be bringing medical supplies—a humanitarian gesture. This triggered the aforementioned: "You'll get this job over my dead body," threat by a commission member, and my, "It's a deal," response.

Unfortunately, our group never made it to North Vietnam. When we arrived in Laos, we learned that President Nixon had decided to bomb Hanoi for the first time. We met with the North Vietnam ambassador who explained that it was not safe to proceed. Understandably, the ambassador didn't want Americans on a human rights mission killed on his watch. He told us that if we left our supplies, he would make sure they got to the Vietnamese medical people.

On July 18, 1972, Haughton announced my appointment retroactive to June 5 (as I had already started my tenure). He also announced the appointment of Bill Silverman, the former director of Michael Reese Hospital, as the new administrative director of County, and Robert Stepto as chair of the department of obstetrics and gynecology. (Silverman, a skilled administrator, safeguarded the interest of the County Board as opposed to the staff in my opinion. My dealings with him were almost always positive. Stepto was a skilled physician and, later, a confidant of my friend Harold Washington.)

The *Tribune* reported that Haughton said, "We are now one big happy family," as he pointed toward Nick Rango.

Nick, whose fate at County was still in the hands of a hearing commission, was quoted as saying, "We applaud the wisdom of the appointments. The two doctors have social vision and clinical skills which we feel will make this the number one public health hospital in the country."

**

Once I settled into my office at County with an administrative staff of four or five, there was no such thing as a typical day, just typical hours—twelve or more. This was a demanding job in both the political and policy sense. I found my new responsibilities so time consuming that they left me with little time for my five children, two of whom were already young adults.

Throughout my life I have been afflicted with "meeting-itis." The condition only got worse when I returned to County. Often I spent half my day in and out of various meetings—with the administration, with other colleagues, and, on occasion with my medical staff. Topics included everything from disciplinary questions to the allocation of resources to choosing staff, and discussing the latest science.

In addition to these scheduled meetings, there were ad hoc gatherings that took place "after hours." Some of the house staff alums remember that when they came by my office during the day, I was almost always on the phone. One of those alums, Gordy Schiff, summarized my style: "Quentin had an open door policy, the door was always open, and he was always on the phone." As I never closed my door, the staffers were privy to at least one side of the conversation if they wanted to stay around and eavesdrop. These same young men and women would regularly congregate around my desk as evening was beginning and the phone calls were ending.

Our discussions were often spirited, as the interns and residents expressed concerns about their patients or registered complaints about the direction of the hospital. They were unhappy that with a snap of his fingers, Haughton had fired some of their colleagues, had forced Gunnar to walk the plank, wanted to drastically reduce their ranks, and had no interest in including them in the decision-making process.

A few more words about the house staff: If a house staff isn't up to snuff in its ability to care for very sick patients, you're going to have a really serious problem at a place like County. We worked very hard to recruit the best doctors available from the U.S. and overseas.

A large number of doctors from abroad—Southeast Asia, India, the Middle East—applied because County was recognized as one of the public hospitals in America that took foreign medical school graduates. It took me a while to learn how to evaluate these applicants. Reading an application, I'd think, *"Gee this guy sounds like the Second Coming, he's really good."* Then one of my colleagues from the attending staff would say, "That university he lists as training is sub-normal. It's like high school." I didn't know that.

I offer that scene to demonstrate the perils of selection. The attending staff was important, but at County in the 1970s, the house staff was the lifeblood of the organization. We put in a lot of time selecting a crew that was well-educated and could understand the American scene. (Of course, just because we accepted someone, foreign or American, didn't mean that he or she came. They could apply to multiple places and some opted to go elsewhere.)

In the end, we did a good job of attracting a classy house staff that would give me great pleasure and occasional headaches over the years. Despite the tenor of the times, medical students in the late 1960s and early 1970s were not that radical. But there were enough committed, progressive would-be interns to fill our seventy openings every year.

Leaping ahead I would say the most significant accomplishment in my tenure at County was that I created a haven where young doctors could come and nourish the talents that would enable them to become leaders in the medical world. Many of these men and women now play leading roles in prison health, occupational health, the treatment of AIDS, the quality standards movement, the community health arena, and other areas.

We were not as successful in recruiting the experienced doctors. Yes, we convinced some accomplished, even celebrated, senior physicians to join us. But many turned down our overtures. Several prominent doctors who were in MCHR came and looked and seriously considered signing on, but at the end of the day we had to do our own recruiting. We had some excellent people to be sure, but it wasn't the easy cascade of scientifically, medically prominent doctors I had hoped for.

Making frequent rounds when you are chief of medicine is not a good idea. A person in a position of authority can breed paranoia among the staff. Doctors and others feel like someone is checking up on them, looking over their shoulders. I tried to keep that to a minimum.

If I wanted to know what was going on with the patients, I went to Ward 35, our medical admitting ward and de facto intensive care unit. It was often the second stop for the patients admitted to the hospital. They went to the ER first.

The people who came into County were sick; only a handful came in for elective surgery or cardiac work-up or the like. As a result, Ward 35, with house and attending staff present, was a busy place, replete with cases that were diagnostically difficult and/or medically complicated.

I'd try to hang around the ward for an hour or two every day, talking to patients as well as doctors to get a feel for what was coming into the medical service. It was during one of these visits that, as I detailed earlier, the elderly patient told me he bypassed so many facilities to come to County because "This is my hospital." As caregivers and caretakers of the public trust, we had an obligation to respect those feelings.

When doctors at County threatened to strike in 1975, I thought they'd be doing a disservice to those who felt "this is my hospital" and to themselves as well. Before talking about that, however, allow me to reflect on some other important initiatives during those years at the hospital.

We can start in the ER. As I explained earlier, when I was doing my own internship and residency at County, we house staffers were assigned shifts in the ER while in the middle of rotations on other wards; there was no separate ER rotation. And there was minimal supervision.

County's ER was as busy and as messy as any ER you've ever seen dramatized on television. There was an endless flow of people, with an endless flow of needs—women who were delivering; people with strokes, heart attacks, appendicitis, victims of stabbings and gun violence. While the residents staffing the ER were skilled and had seen a great deal in their time at the hospital, they were not to be confused with fully trained certified doctors.

When I returned to County, I found a functioning ER in need of an upgrade. Still staffed by residents plucked from the wards, it was too haphazard. So, as I recall, we did two things: we made the ER part of the rotation and we placed attendings in the ER.

Under this new system residents spent thirty days straight in ER, rather than, say, a day or two a month. And attendings could now begin to specialize in emergency medicine. County had one of the earliest trauma units in the country, circa 1966. Staffed by doctors who knew their business, the ER became a refuge for the hundreds of thousands of Chicago-area patients who relied on it.

While not the stuff of prime-time viewing, another initiative was also critical: We updated patient records so that third parties could be billed. Believe it or not, County, in perpetual fiscal distress, had not previously done this. As a result there were significant sums of uncollected receivables on the books—receivables that, if collected, could be used to make the hospital a better place.

Many patients had insurance from their jobs. Blacks in particular were not accepted in other hospitals and despite their employment their insurance was not effectively billed at County. Others received Medicare or Medicaid. Yet there had not been an orderly system for billing and collecting from insurance companies or the government. Previous administrations had, for the most part, failed to charge for services that these third parties were obliged to pay.

It seemed like common sense to get all the money that was due for services rendered. I insisted that the doctors in my department cooperate by keeping up-to-date records and validating whether they did or did not do particular services—procedures, injections, and a variety of things that doctors do that are compensable. As a result we collected over half a million dollars in receivables.

Occupational health was another initiative of which I'm very proud. Shortly after becoming chief of medicine, I was approached by Dr. Bert Carnow. We had been in practice together some years earlier. Then he had departed to establish a practice with a heavy emphasis on workmen's compensation cases. We had a somewhat stormy relationship prior to 1972, and it would become even stormier over the coming years. But to Bert's credit, he was an early champion of occupational and environmental issues and had helped establish the Occupational Health Department at the School of Public Health at University of Illinois-Chicago, where we were both on the faculty.

Bert proposed to me that UIC and County develop a combined program that would add an extra year of occupational medicine training to our existing internal medicine training program. Those who completed the training and passed an exam would then become board certified in occupational health *and* internal medicine.

This was an enterprising and unique proposal, and the timing was perfect. In 1970, Congress had passed the Occupation Safety and Health Act, which, among other things, created the Occupational Safety and Health Administration (OSHA). MCHR, which had moved its national office from Philadelphia to Chicago in 1972, was beginning to expand its efforts beyond civil rights to a variety of public health issues, including occupational health, thanks to the leadership of Don Wharton, Phyllis Cullen, and David Wegman. The unions in Chicago and elsewhere were also becoming increasingly involved in fighting for occupational safety.

At this time almost all the occupational health professionals were working for industry, not for the workers and the unions. Excited by the prospect of leveling the playing field by developing a cadre of physicians committed to worker safety and health, I made the necessary arrangements on the organizational side to create this program.

Was that difficult? It's hard to exaggerate, but even in a work environment where the politicos didn't particularly like me, the power of a chair of medicine or surgery is enormous. There is a lot of authority built into that post. I submitted a proposal with a budget for a new department of occupational medicine, and it was approved. We then announced that we would be accepting applications for a program that would prepare participants for a masters in public health and board certification in internal medicine and occupational medicine.

The occupational health program began in 1976. With four students in each year's class, we eventually had sixteen participants at any given time—the largest program of its kind in the country. Our graduates went on to have distinguished careers in the field, working for non-governmental organizations (NGOs), the government, medical practices, and corporations. (Sadly, in the face of a budgetary crisis in 2007, the Division of Occupational Medicine was eliminated along with some clinics. Led by Dr. Peter Orris, an early County trainee, there is interest today in reconstituting the department if resources can be found.)

Around the same time that we launched the academic program a coalition of medical professionals, labor leaders, and others created the Chicago Area Committee on Occupational Safety and Health (CACOSH). This first of its kind alliance included the regional United Steel Workers, the regional United Auto Workers, and the regional Oil Chemical and Atomic Workers, whose legislative director, Tony Mazzocchi, was a major force in the occupational safety and health movement.

The effort was designed to fit the needs of any union willing to work with its membership on health and safety issues. Health professionals and students provided education and research. By design the coalition was under the union leadership.

Chicago was now the center of the national occupational health movement. Bob Johnson of the Chicago area UAW and I were the leaders of the local chapter. Within two or three years, our model had spread across the country, with twenty chapters. The movement spawned many workplace improvements—such as workers' rights to know about the chemicals they are working with—that are now enshrined in national law.

Revamping our relationship with the pharmaceutical companies was also a front-burner initiative at County. Then as now, the drug companies had a powerful influence over the conduct of doctors. We like to think of ourselves as independent, scientifically motivated and guided, but the fact is that the pharmaceutical industry has an army of skilled salesmen who have all sorts of blandishments to encourage you that their wares are the answer to your patients' problems—in particular their company's trademarked, costly drugs as opposed to no drugs or drugs that are simpler and less costly.

Our doctors were routinely prescribing pills—most notably

tranquilizers and sedatives—to far too many of the thousands of patients a day who came to the outpatient clinic. Of course, these drugs have a place in treating insomnia and other conditions, but they should not be the default approach to the exclusion of spending time with the patient and determining if a non-pharmaceutical response is better. It was time to just say no to over-prescribing tranquilizers and sedatives and drugs that mask symptoms.

We made a rule that in the outpatient clinic, house staff orders for tranquilizers had to be countersigned by attending physicians. That sounds like it's inhibiting, maybe even insulting, but interns and residents are doctors in training. We wanted their training to deal with the fact that there are other answers to medical problems besides drugs. We wanted our doctors to empathize and talk to their patients and when necessary give them medication, but not just automatically write some sedating prescription.

Result? It was projected that on a yearly basis one million fewer prescriptions were written for restricted drugs.

In addition to restricting drugs, we wanted to restrict drug salesmen. My "aha moment" came during a meeting with my chief residents. (There were perhaps a dozen chief residents in the fourteen wards that the Department of Medicine controlled.) We were having a discussion in the lobby of the interns' quarters. Nearby the drug salesmen were noisily hawking their drugs to other residents.

We asked the salesmen for quiet. Ha! They were so arrogant that they laughed at the request. That was a mistake. It stimulated my resolve to have control over them, so we initiated a revolutionary new policy. We changed the relationship between these vendors and our residents and attendings. The salesmen could no longer go on the wards. They couldn't interrupt doctors when they were doing their regular duties. They had to make appointments at fixed times to meet the doctors if they wanted to extol to them the virtues of their drugs.

Looking back on these times I'm proud of another initiative: helping facilitate the appointment of Dr. Jerry Moss as chair of County's Department of Surgery. Moss was a gifted surgeon. We didn't see the world the same way—he was far more conservative than I—but we respected each other. As chairs of the hospital's two biggest departments, we worked well together. Later he became dean at the School of Medicine at UIC.

These various initiatives seemed to please Haughton and the administration. Judith Barnard's *Chicago* magazine article reminds me that between 1972 and 1975, I received three evaluations. There were twelve categories on each evaluation, and I was given the top mark in each category, each year. Over that period I was also given raises that brought my salary up to about $60,000.

So why, in the fall of 1975, did Jim Haughton fire me? And why, when a federal judge reinstated me, did Jim fire me again?

Ten

On November 26, 1975, the day before Thanksgiving, Jim Haughton handed me a one-page memorandum notifying me that I was fired. "These things are never easy," he said.

I shook my head. "I'm the one who's getting fired. Why?" The memo, which ordered me to leave my office by 5 p.m., offered no explanation.

Jim, with hospital director Bill Silverman at his side, told me that they didn't have to give me a reason, adding that I was so high up in the hierarchy of employees that I could be dismissed without any explanation.

"I don't think that's true," I said. I was bluffing. I didn't know the law. "I don't like this and I think the staff and the patients in my department need me. I'm not going to give up my post." Again I asked, "Why are you firing me?"

Jim continued to refuse to give a reason for my termination. But it wasn't hard to read between the lines.

One month earlier, on October 27, the hospital's house staff had gone on strike. While I had not endorsed this tactic, I had endorsed the staff's demands—the vast majority of which focused on patient care. I had been critical of Haughton and the commission during the work stoppage. Indeed, I had even joined others in calling for the ouster of the commission because it had failed to fulfill its duties under the law. If a department head was going to roll post-strike, it was surely going to be mine.

While I could figure out the motive for my firing, I was, nevertheless, surprised. The strike had been settled on November 17.

There was a relatively warm feeling in our hospital community. I thought the powers that be, though bitter about the stoppage, were happy with the amicable settlement—a settlement that I still take great pride in helping to have fashioned. I hadn't done anything insubordinate. Rather, I'd done my best to hold the operation together during the strike—with some success—and push for a resolution.

Recently a portion of Judith Barnard's article in *Chicago* magazine was brought to my attention: "At the height of the strike an intern had said to Haughton in the hall one day, 'How does it feel, Dr. Haughton, to have the press against you, the doctors against you, the patients against you, and a lot of your own staff against you?' And Haughton had said, 'No one is against me except Quentin Young.'"

And I thought we were friends.

The timing of my dismissal was interesting. According to one HHGC commissioner, the decision to fire me was made on November 14, but was not immediately announced. Three days later the house staff voted to ratify the new contract, thereby ending their strike. And nine days after that I was formally handed my pink slip.

Is it possible that Haughton and the commission feared that firing me before the vote would have alienated those casting ballots and resulted in continuation of the strike? We can only speculate. But consider the actions the house staff took immediately after hearing I'd been fired. As the *Tribune* reported: "(They) voted not to take any disruptive action, but decided to post a 24-hour guard outside Young's office to assure nothing would be done to deny him access. Several young doctors removed a door to Young's inner office so it could not be locked."

At the same time, "During a noisy session, the hospital's senior staff—including chairmen of all major departments—voiced unanimous support for Young and condemned his firing." The headline (and dark humor) here is that the senior staff rarely, if ever, supported anything unanimously.

My response to the brouhaha was simple. "I plan to remain at my post until given my constitutional rights to a hearing, and

I'm sure I'll be vindicated," I announced. And that's what I did until that hearing, albeit at desks other than my own. My nomadic existence was occasioned by the administration's decision to put a door back on my office—and padlock it.

So how did we come to the strike, my firing, and, as we shall see, my vindication and then a second firing?

Hospitals were not immune to the political activism of the 1960s and '70s. In March of 1975, the Committee of Interns and Residents of New York City went on strike at 21 hospitals. They returned to work four days later after the hospitals agreed to eliminate every-other-night work schedules. County's approximately 450 interns and residents had also formed what was, in effect, their own collective bargaining unit, the House Staff Association (HSA).

Negotiations between HSA and the commission began early in 1975. It's interesting to note that few of the staff's 100-plus demands were intended to benefit them directly. As I recall they weren't threatening to strike for an increase in pay or more time off or better working conditions. They wanted such things as more staffing, more nurses, better equipment, streamlined procedures, better processing of lab tests, and interpreters for the increasing number of Spanish-speaking patients.

Here's one demand I still remember, a demand that gets to the heart of HSA's primarily altruistic thrust. When a newly-admitted patient was brought to a ward, the lights had to be turned on throughout the entire ward. There was no way of just turning on localized lights near the patient's bed. As a result the whole ward—some eighty folks—would be awakened by a fully-lit late night or early morning admission. Unnecessary 3 a.m. wake-ups are not healthy for sick people, so the house staff wanted bedside lamps for the patients.

Oh the audacity, the foolhardiness. What were these upstarts thinking by focusing their demands on the betterment of the patient instead of themselves?

Writes Barnard: "The house staff called it 'simple, basic demands to benefit the patients by bringing the hospital up to AMA standards.' Haughton called it an attempt 'by the youngest, least experienced members of the staff to dictate the policies of the hospital.'.... Dr. Samuel Hoffman, head of the Hektoen Research Institute at County, called it 'an attempt by the Communists to take over the hospital and eventually the country.'"

I called it a timely and reasonable demand.

Despite the activism of the times, in 1975 a well-organized house staff was an unusual animal. Over the preceding twenty or thirty years, County's interns and residents had periodically attempted to establish what you could describe as a union. But because house staffs are by nature transient, such organizing is inherently difficult. Interns may only be around for a year. Residents will stay for three or perhaps up to five years. So unless you are one of the handful of young doctors that will be joining the attending staff, you are most likely passing through while getting credentialed. You are not necessarily fully invested in the future of the institution you will soon be leaving.

At County, which boasted so many different specialties, the more active house staff unionists were in medicine and pediatrics and family practice. Trainees in surgery and surgical specialties were less interested. I've never done a formal study, but I think this is because the people who go into surgery are in general more conservative than those in primary care.

By October, agreement had been reached on many issues, mostly those related to employment. Still unresolved, however, were many demands related to patient care. When the staff overwhelmingly rejected what Haughton presented as his last, best offer, the strike was on.

I've been asked many times if I was consulted by the HSA. Or if Haughton asked me to exert some kind of influence on them not to organize like they did. Or if I was just a passive observer.

To understand my role, keep in mind that I was an atypical chief of service. The typical head of a major medical or surgical service at County was a physician who was career-oriented. I brought to my post a different certain set of objectives. I wanted very much to get the health services of the county into the community, to broaden the type of service we offered, to go beyond just dealing with emergencies or problems that were already developed and address prevention through better nutrition, immunization, control of chronic disease, and other means.

To achieve this I needed a strong medical staff. Many of the seventy interns per year that were attracted to the program—some, because of my reputation—had a certain political bent. They were new medical school graduates who came specifically because of the public sector mission in Chicago and to make this public hospital more responsive to its patients' needs. These young doctors and I were on the same wavelength. The paradox here, however, was that I was not one of the team; I was the boss. I was *their* boss.

Some of the things they wanted were not compatible with what I wanted. By and large, however, I felt that the house staff's demands were reasonable and would be beneficial to patients and the hospital. Moreover, the fact that the house staff itself was taking an initiative was very significant. Across the United States, house staffs were not participants in these kind of planning services.

But I need to dispel some myths. I was not the hand behind the house staff organization. I knew the leaders and liked them a lot. I had encouraged them to come to County, and they were good doctors. They wanted the environment to improve, which would mean clashing with the administration. As chair of medicine, I was different from most of the administration in that I supported most of their demands and criticisms. Nonetheless, during the preceding years and the years that would follow, the well-intentioned house staff and their well-intentioned chair of medicine (me) would butt heads on occasion.

The HSA didn't include attending physicians or department heads. When the house staffers made their decision to strike, they didn't come and ask my advice. They came to tell me what they had in mind. (Once that decision was made, I believed that it would be good if we could resolve the dispute in a way that would improve conditions for the doctors and the patients going forward. If the house staff lost the strike, our ability to recruit and keep good doctors would be much harder.)

By now you might be asking yourself if it's a good idea for doctors to go on strike at a hospital. By stopping work aren't they jeopardizing the health and well-being of the patients? Patients whose health and well-being is supposedly the impetus for the strike? After all, ceasing to provide medical care is quite different than ceasing to produce automobiles or pack meat (not that striking private industry isn't also justified).

The house staff recognized this. As a result they announced that while they would stop admitting and treating patients, they would be available in the event the non-union attending doctors filling their shoes were overwhelmed with work.

While I applauded this concession as well as the HSA demands, I nevertheless offered my unsolicited two cents worth that a strike against a public hospital was a dangerous tactic. In so many words I said: *You almost certainly enjoy respect and support from the public for the hard work that you do and the fact that you need equipment that isn't there. But if in the course of your strike, heaven forbid, one or more people die or suffer life-threatening setbacks, the public—your supporters—will find it very hard to absolve you. You strikers will be blamed.*

If you want to measure how much influence I had on the HSA, consider that my advice was ignored.

While dealing with the HSA was at times difficult, the commission and Haughton were far more exasperating. Jim and I met one-on-one frequently during the weeks leading up to the strike, and I repeatedly told him he could avoid a stoppage by meeting HSA's modest, reasonable demands regarding patient care. Along with others, I also urged him to name an attending physician to the administration's negotiating team. We felt that such a person could bridge the gap between the administration and the HSA and resolve the matter quickly. Request denied. The governing commission—meaning Haughton—said, *Oh no, we couldn't do that because that would compromise the future relationship between attendings and house staff.*

Why was Haughton so unyielding? I'm guessing here, but I suspect he was receiving counsel and encouragement from the Chicago-based American Hospital Association to hold firm against the militant young doctors, to break the union's back. I believe, although I have no proof of this, that the events at County were closely monitored by the Hospital Association because house staff organizing in a variety of hospitals across the country was on the rise.

The Hospital Association wanted very much for Haughton to break this strike. Its idea of a good doctor was one who was totally subordinate and subservient to the administration. Because of such outside pressure or simply because he desired to maintain his own institutional authority, Haughton ignored my argument that he would become a hero in the world of health care training and health care delivery if he reached an equitable settlement with the house staff.

The leadership of the hospital was playing with fire—aka the well-being of patients—by taking such a hard line to assert their power. Worse, it was fanning the flames by repeated public pronouncements that County was still open for business, that patients should keep on coming if and when a strike started. In my opinion, this was irresponsible, dangerous. You can't lose several hundred house staff and take care of the people who are already in beds, much less newly admitted patients. If your goal is to solve the problem of health care, don't overload a system that is already operating beyond its capacity.

But what did I know? Apparently the governing commission felt that continuing to admit patients was a smart tactic that would scare the house staff into returning lest an innocent patient die. What a game of brinksmanship to play for seventeen days.

Within the hospital we had an executive medical committee of about thirty, composed of the leaders of all the different departments. This committee had to confront this unusual situation of no house staff working. Many of us joined the non-striking attending physicians and threw ourselves into caring for patients.

Day One of the strike wasn't too bad. Day Two was a bit worse. After a week or ten days, those of us on duty were tired. We didn't get to work our shift and go to bed. We had to stay on call.

Meanwhile, the house staff kept its promise to help when called upon. On those occasions when we'd have an influx of sick people, we would tell the strikers and they'd send people over to help. This was not the ideal dynamic. By and large the house staff is subordinate to the attending staff and to have to ask them or even implore them to give us some help made for disarray or at least discontent among the attendings, who increasingly had to do the job of the striking house staff.

What did the patients think of all this? Patients at County, and maybe patients elsewhere as well, didn't have any sense of authority or power. They didn't think they could order people to or from anywhere. To the extent they chose sides, I think their sympathies were with the house staff, the worker bees. As previously mentioned, the typical patient felt County was the place where the best doctors were and where the best care was delivered despite the often decrepit facilities. I didn't hear any complaints about or criticism of the strike. To the best of my knowledge, the patients just accepted it as part of their daily reality.

As for the general public? To this day I think the strike was a dangerous gamble. People die at County Hospital all the time for obvious reasons. You would think that this would have been exacerbated by the strike. Happily that wasn't the case, so there was no tragedy to raise the blood pressure of the average man or woman on the street.

I didn't spend a lot of time surveying people's opinion, but in general my own circle of friends was supportive. Like me, they worried that with one strike-related patient death, this could go terribly wrong. This said, as the strike continued, the patience of my friends, the public, and even those of us working hard in the hospital waned. We all wanted the strike to end.

On the day the strike began, the governing commission went to court. Cook County Circuit Court Judge Donald J. O'Brien granted its motion for an injunction that limited the number of picketers at each entrance to the hospital. Eventually, some strikers would be jailed ignoring the injunction.

The judge, who was not sympathetic to the HSA, also offered to mediate the strike. The commission refused. To me, this was a clear sign that the commission was not operating in good faith; they wanted the strike to be broken, not negotiated. (A few days later, the commission also rejected the Reverend Jesse Jackson's offer to mediate.)

During the first week of the strike, my colleague Jorge Prieto, head of the hospital's Department of Family Medicine, and I held a press conference. There we fired our first shots at the commission. Allow attending physicians to join the negotiations, we said. No, said the commission.

Those negotiations had stopped five days before the strike began. They finally resumed—sans attending physicians—with federal mediators on Day Ten of the stoppage. The commission remained intransigent. And so, the executive medical staff took a bold step.

The law that created the governing commission included a provision for recalling members for just cause—failure to perform their duties or to show up for meetings—all the reasons you have for replacing leaders of a board. Aware of this, the executive medical staff sent a letter to the "Selectors" who had the authority to choose members of the governing commission. In effect the executive medical staff said, the governing commission was guilty of "misconduct and malfeasance" in not fulfilling its responsibility of providing care to the people for whom it is responsible, namely poor people without insurance. Per the law, we wanted the governing commission to be recalled and replaced.

On Day 13 of the strike, a handful of fellow executive medical staff members and I met with the selectors to press our case. And what happened? Quickly the situation changed. We had found the Achilles heel of the governing commission: the fear of recall by the selection committee. The governing commission agreed to put four senior physicians on the negotiating team. Among them was Jack Saletta, assistant chair of the Department of Surgery. Within a few days the parties had reached an agreement.

The commission didn't give away the store. That was never in the cards. As my friend Ron Shansky, a junior attending physician, said in the *Chicago* magazine article, "The house staff were always willing to compromise. It wasn't so important that they didn't get all the patient care items they wanted. What was important was the right to be a part of patient care decisions."

I agree. In a public hospital like Cook County, the house staff has a much greater responsibility than house staff in private hospitals. By and large their work-load is heavier than residents in private hospitals, and the imperfection in equipment and administration make their difficult tasks harder. It was appropriate, even laudable that these young doctors indicated the unmet needs of their patients.

You may have sensed that I am not always one to let sleeping dogs lie. This was the case after the strike. On November 20, I joined a few other doctors in sending a letter to John Sengstacke, the publisher of the *Chicago Defender* and chairman of the selection committee. We again pressed our case that the governing commission be dismissed for, among other things: risking the well-being of patients by continuing to admit patients during the strike over the protests of the overworked, increasingly fatigued doctors who remained on duty, refusing to control or monitor (Haughton) during the strike and hereafter, and refusing to permit executive staff members to participate in the strike negotiations.

The decision to fire me may have been made during the strike, but this letter surely didn't help matters. Helping my spirits was the outpouring of support from unexpected as well as expected parties. The sentiments of the door-removing house staff were echoed by chair of surgery Jerry Moss and Dr. Vincent Collins, president of the hospital's medical staff. As the *Tribune* reported, Collins called my firing "appalling and incredible. I think it's leading toward catastrophe." He also predicted that med school grads would now be discouraged from applying for internships at County. Finally, he said that firing me violated hospital bylaws that mandated hearings before dismissal of staff doctors. My point exactly.

A December 1st editorial in the *Tribune* also argued that I was entitled to a hearing. It then added: "Instead of peremptorily dismissing Dr. Young, the Governing Commission should attempt a serious and substantial reply to the charges Dr. Young and the other staff doctors have brought. It should show respect for the dignity of its own major administrative positions and for at least some of its adversaries."

I love the way Judith Barnard describes the days that followed:

"Within the next few weeks, the most conservative physicians in America would begin to sound like the liberal wing of the ACLU. Young had become the symbol of the tenuous relationship of top executives to the top executive—one not limited to but especially crucial in hospitals where the problem of shared responsibility takes on profound implications for the rest of the population who may literally live or die by the way these executives and their staffs function."

Conservative physicians, as you've come to read on the preceding pages, equals the AMA. Though still a member, I was hardly enamored of the organization. Nor was the AMA a fan of me. But the story was becoming bigger than Quentin Young or the house staff strike; this had to do with the rights of doctors and the governance of hospitals.

Having retained a lawyer to assure that I had my day in court, I received word that a committee of the AMA's local branch, the Chicago Medical Society, was preparing to vote 3-2 to verbally support my reinstatement, but not to contribute to my legal defense—a defense that we knew would run in the tens of thousands of dollars. What? I called the AMA and said something like, *You guys are crazy. I didn't ask for your support, I didn't want it. But to take the position that you won't back me financially is like saying you think I'm guilty. And it's not me. It's doctors' rights in any given hospital situation.*

The AMA invited me to press my case at a council meeting before the vote. Recovering from hernia surgery, I went reluctantly. I was polite and diplomatic, but in effect I said, *You guys are jerks and go to hell.* Such flattery did the trick! They voted to give me $15,000, and from that point forward, they were quite supportive.

My lawyer Dick Watt explained to me that we had to make several decisions. Should I take the initiative and go to court to request a hearing to determine if my firing was justified? Or should I continue working and wait to see if the commission went to court to get me out for good? I had already been denied access to my office and administrative staff. I wasn't being paid and my insurance had been rescinded. As the attendings had been ordered not to accompany me on rounds, I saw patients with some seventy supportive interns in tow. Dr. George Dunea was appointed to replace me and take my title as chair of medicine.

And then the final straw. They took my parking space. That did it. I held a press conference in the parking lot. "They shouldn't fire me," I told reporters.

After deciding I was better off going to court rather than waiting for the commission to do so, I had to determine whether state or federal court would be best. Watt told me that if we went to state court I would probably win; the court would say I could not be fired prior to a hearing in accordance with the hospital bylaws. But, he added, the process might take a year or more.

Federal court would be faster, he said. But my odds of prevailing in that venue would be about 50/50. My fate, Watt suggested, would depend on whether we got a randomly assigned judge who was liberal or conservative. Neither my supporters nor I had the fire in the belly to drag this affair out a year, nor for that matter did my enemies. We'd take our chances in federal court with a suit charging that the firing without a hearing had violated my civil rights.

As fate would have it, we drew U.S. District Court Judge Bernard Decker, a no-nonsense Republican who had been appointed by President John F. Kennedy. On our first visit to the courtroom, two weeks after I'd been fired, we watched as Judge Decker sentenced two public officials who had been found guilty of taking bribes. He looked down from the bench with contempt and told the fellows that he was sick and tired of government corruption.

Now it was our turn. Up stood Tom Foran, the attorney for the governing commission. (The same Tom Foran, who as U.S. Attorney, had prosecuted the Chicago Seven.) With great certainty he argued that I had no standing in the court. He cited a statute that he said authorized the commission to fire department heads like me sans hearing for any reason it chose.

Judge Decker retired to his chambers. Returning a short time later, the judge said he could not find the statute Foran had cited. The reason he couldn't find it was simple. That cited statute, which did indeed allow for a dismissal without recourse, had been superseded by the state legislature.

My lawyer knew that, but he didn't let the court know immediately. Instead, he let Foran hem and haw for a bit. Finally, he rose and said, "Your Honor, I think I can help here." Judge Decker barked at him to sit down. Getting nowhere with our adversary, the judge eventually allowed Watt to speak. "That used to be the case," he explained, "but the law has been repealed and replaced with a law that affords people like Dr. Young due process."

I thought Judge Decker was going to kill Foran. Better than that, he said I was entitled to a hearing and reinstated me. He then told the commission if it wanted to try and oust me, it should file formal charges against me. At that point he'd appoint an independent fact-finding panel.

When I returned to County, I was no longer a man without a department or an office. But as expected, a few weeks later in mid-January, the commission filed those formal charges, alleging that I had abetted the strike. Judge Decker then appointed a three-person fact-finding panel, which in March held twelve days of hearings.

On April 3, 1976, the panel announced its findings. In its opinion I had violated hospital rules by getting involved in the strike negotiations contrary to the orders of my bosses. However, the panel continued, in doing so I had been acting in good faith to ensure that our patients received the best possible care. Dismissal was not justified, it said. The panel did recommend that I be suspended without pay for thirty days and that a reprimand be put in my personnel file.

You might think the commission would accept the findings of the court-ordered panel and move forward. Instead, on April 30, the commission fired me again. By a vote of 5 to 3, I was given my second pink slip. The three dissenters urged that the panel's recommendations be accepted.

My reaction was swift. "I think tonight that the commissioners who voted to fire me attempted to act as the executioners of the hospital," I said. County's executive medical staff called for the firing of the five commissioners who had voted to fire me. Vincent Collins was quoted in the *Tribune* as saying that staff morale was "at the lowest ebb that I believe it could possibly be. I can't believe that so-called reasonable men could be so vindictive."

My lawyers responded by saying they would ask Judge Decker to review the decision. He did, and in late May he ruled that the commission had exceeded its power in firing me. Moreover, he permanently enjoined them from firing me on these charges—a kind of double jeopardy ruling. As the *Tribune* reported, "Decker said he hoped there would be no more litigation and the two sides would 'put aside the hostilities of last year's strike and work together.' Young's firing resulted in 'bitter controversy that has polarized and disrupted the hospital' and has been viewed by some 'as part of a power struggle for control over Cook County Hospital,' Decker said."

I wasn't ready to put aside my hostility. "Young back in job, hits at hospital," ran a headline in the next day's *Tribune*. In the newspaper's words, I "continued the war by challenging the commissioners to put more outpatient facilities in neighborhoods." I added that the commissioners were not equipped to make the critical decisions here. "The commission (members) have administrators with no background in health care delivery. The medical staff does. The question is, are they (the commissioners) going to continue the fiction that we are there as their handmaidens."

After I was reinstated for the second time, I announced, "I'm certainly not going to make a decision now publicly about my future. I have some personal notions about public interest and health policy."

As it turned out I would continue at County longer than the governing commission itself would survive. But there was a more important question concerning survival: Would a crumbling, financially strapped Cook County Hospital continue to live or would it be shuttered—its patients dispersed to hospitals that didn't want them?

Linda Rae Murray

Linda Rae Murray was a resident at Cook County Hospital in internal medicine and occupational medicine from 1977-1980. Over the past three decades she has continued to work with Dr. Young on a wide range of issues and organizations including the American Public Health Association and the board of Health and Medicine Policy Research Group.

Quentin is a Chicago fixture. When I arrived in Chicago in 1966 to attend college, it was not long before Dr. Young's name came up in a variety of settings. In the summer before classes started Dr. King was struck by a rock leading a demonstration through Marquette Park. Quentin was his physician. The campus was abuzz with anti-Vietnam war activities. Quentin's name would be mentioned. Some movement person would fall ill with no money... go and see Dr. Young. The Medical Committee for Human Rights, and its role in providing medical support for important demonstrations, (e.g. 1968 Democratic Party Convention) got my attention and always Quentin was there.

But I must admit, an "old" white doc (several years older than my parents) did not capture sustained attention of a young Black radical. Little did I realize in those early years how Quentin would intertwine with my life and profoundly affect my professional career.

In those first years in Chicago, I had no plans to enter medicine. But all over the city, among movement activists, Dr. Young had a solid reputation. He was someone who could be depended upon; high praise for a white guy.

I entered medical school as a daughter of my community, a participant in our struggle. I was guided by Black physicians, housekeepers, teachers, and steel workers but I did not yet fully appreciate the peculiar institution called American Medicine.

In medical school I met three physicians who helped shape my understanding of the failures of health care in American. Dr. Jorge Prieto, who would chair the Department of Family Medicine at County, was straightforward in his advice to young students of color. " Being a doctor is a privilege and you are obligated to speak up for those who cannot and fight for justice for all." Jorge practiced in the community and helped County establish community based health centers. Dr. Prieto, a Mexican immigrant, understood racism and worked for unity of Blacks and Latinos in an effort to increase the numbers of minority health professionals. Dr. Bertram Carnow (an old practice partner of Quentin's) introduced me to occupational health and how workplace toxins so often destroyed the health and lives of workers. Bert would establish at Cook County Hospital a residency in Occupational Medicine.

Of course there was Quentin. He sat in our school's Department of Preventive Medicine. He offered a clear understanding of the failures of American Medicine. He established a successful Urban Preceptorship for medical students, showing us the warts of the system and more importantly how to change things. "Everything, poverty, housing, jobs, racism... everything impacts the health of your patients." This was Quentin's message.

As a medical student I carefully watched the activities across the street at County Hospital. Quentin was recruited to County in a desperate effort to help save the hospital. Our teachers in medical school were adamant... "STAY AWAY FROM COUNTY!" A strike of the house staff insisting on better conditions for their patients. Quentin supported the demands. "STAY AWAY FROM COUNTY" A conference sponsored by MCHR spawned the first COSH (Committee for Occupational Safety and Health) group in the nation (CACOSH). Quentin was part of its leadership.

I was about to choose my residency. I wanted to practice in the Black community, among people abused by American medicine. But I was unsure of exactly what to do, or for that matter what area of medicine to pursue. There was a "missionary" spirit of many young white residents at County that distressed Black & Latino students and house staff. Did I really want to spend those critical years with a bunch of white missionaries who viewed my community, and me for that matter, as an exotic adventure? I weighed the possibility of getting good training at County. Perhaps I should listen (for once) to the voice of authority and train somewhere else. I could hear my great-grandmother admonishing me to remember that if you are Black, "you have to be twice as good to get half as much." After all, I had the rest of my career to practice in the Black community.

Then a classmate came to me excited...; "Linda, County is starting a residency in that program you are interested in." What? I was still trying to decide between pediatrics and internal medicine... what program could they mean? "You know, the one about what makes workers sick." Perfect timing. Bert Carnow was starting in Quentin's department a joint residency in Occupational Medicine and Internal Medicine. Dr. Carnow had pieced together support from unions, the Governing Commission and Dr. Young to start his residency. Dr. Prieto was spending his time at County forcing them to branch out to community medicine and to respond to the rapidly growing Latino population. And Quentin David Young M.D. was holding down the fort doing battle with a corrupt Chicago machine and winning improvements in health care for the county's poor. When the time came to fill out the computer matching system used to place medical students in residency programs, I filled in just one institution... Cook County Hospital.

Quentin's years at County were never dull. The departments of

160

medicine and family practice had more than their share of idealistic activists. Members of many political left organizations from the Communist Party, the RCP (Revolutionary Communist Party), Black Panthers to name a few were part of the house staff. There was a militant house staff union and nurses union, and an active Black House staff Organization. The hospital reflected the times. The County was in crisis and hospital workers joined with community activists in a struggle to save County Hospital. Dr. Young was our boss. As any good trade unionist will tell you... a boss is a boss is a boss. Dr. Young tried to give advice and provide guidance to the many "youngsters" dedicated to fighting for the hospital. We listened (sort of)... but this was some OLD WHITE DOCTOR who was our BOSS. We ignored him whenever we felt like it. During my tenure as the president of the House Staff Association we had the relationship you might expect between a boss and a union activist. We clashed over how to influence the Governing Commission, we clashed over the best way to get better health care for the County Jail inmates, we clashed over how to guarantee good educational experiences for house staff. We had arguments of methods and tactics, never differences of goals and principle.

Quentin left County before my residency ended. His departure signaled a new period of decline for the institution. No department head in the past thirty plus years has accomplished as much as Quentin was able to do during his tenure.

All teenagers are amazed at how much their parents learn in the decades after the teens leave home. So it was with me and Quentin. It was impossible to escape him. I worked with him on campaign after campaign. He provided leadership in organizations where I held membership. He spoke out on issues that I cared about. He served on Harold Washington's Board of Health, he was president of PNHP and APHA. Today he serves as Chair of HMPRG. We continue to work as colleagues over the many decades that followed our time together at County Hospital.

Choosing to do my residency under Quentin at Cook County Hospital changed my life. I am a product of Quentin's residency, I am one of his professional children. His style of medicine penetrated the entire department, his work ethic, his optimism, and his joy of caring for patients was imprinted on "his children." His day to day work merged his high quality technical practice of clinical medicine with his insistence on fighting racism and injustice. Before Quentin, I had envisioned my career as a physician being my nine to five; saving my struggle for justice for after work hours. During the County years Quentin seamlessly went from rounds to case discussions to phone conversations with reporters. He showed us that there was no way to practice medicine without including the fight to improve all of the conditions of life and society that make our patients healthy or sick.

He has never missed a beat; he continues to fight for the things we both believe in. He continues today, to demonstrate how to carve a unified life of struggle making no false separation between career, family and the struggle for social justice. He continues to devote time to teaching the young, creating more health workers who understand that the struggle for social justice is not an extracurricular activity but the foundations of our professional work.

Quentin is twenty-five years my senior. I hope to accomplish half as much in my next twenty five years as he has done in the past twenty five years. But whatever I do in the future I will welcome his laugh, the twinkle in his eye, his fierce commitment to justice and especially his advice on the next steps we must take.

Eleven

In 1976, the community and the staff at County had more to worry about than my future as chief of medicine. The future of the hospital itself was up in the air. What was the matter? What wasn't? There were problems with governance, the budget, the delivery of services, and a crumbling physical plant.

And so was born the Committee to Save Cook County Hospital. As my friend Dr. Linda Rae Murray, the president of the House Staff, explained in 1979 when the situation was even more dire: "Our committee was formed… out of the concern of its patients, staff members, and a significant spectrum of community organizations for the hospital's future. Inadequate County Board budget allotments and lagging state support for the hospital's services to the medically indigent have year by year forced serious cutbacks in its personnel and services."

It's worth spending a little time here to talk about Linda and two other house staff members who were instrumental in creating the Committee, the husband and wife team of Dr. Gordy Schiff and Dr. Mardge Cohen. All three came up through the ranks when I was chief of medicine and, along with others too numerous to mention, have become national leaders in health and medicine committed to helping the needy. I look upon them as my second set of children, and I am as proud of them as I am of my own five kids.

Linda, who hailed from Cleveland, had earned her MD from the University of Illinois-Chicago in 1977. She then came to County for her residency. There, she was elected head of the

House Staff. After completing her residency and earning a masters in Public Health, she left County in 1981 to work in Canada and then teach at Meharry, a traditionally black medical school in Memphis.

In 1979, a BBC film crew came to County to do a documentary about health care in urban America. (More details about this later.) The documentary's title, "I CALL IT MURDER," was a quotation from Linda about the systematic shunting of the poor to County Hospital from all corners of the community.

In the film, Linda acknowledged that she could be making three times as much money in private practice, but felt a strong moral obligation to work in the public health field. She has been true to those words for the last thirty-plus years, and today serves as Chief Medical Officer of the Cook County Department of Health. She is also an adjunct professor at the University of Illinois at Chicago School of Public Health and sees patients as a general internist at the Woodlawn Health Center on Chicago's South Side.

During her training period and after, Linda used the hospital to buffer the paucity of care with a hard working medical staff. The dumping of the sick poor by other hospitals gave indigent people a place to go, but allowed private hospitals a way to get out of taking care of the uninsured. Linda fought to get County adequately funded and staffed, while she and others strove to make the sixty-plus hospitals in Chicago take responsibility for contributing to the care of the sick poor.

Gordy Schiff, a general internist, came to County after graduating from Rush Medical College in 1976. Already devoted to the hospital from his summers volunteering in the Emergency Room as a pre-med student in the early '

'70s, he stayed for three decades, directing the General Medicine Clinic and chairing the hospital's Quality Assurance/Quality Improvement Committee, among other things. At the same time he was on the faculty at Rush.

In 2007, he joined the Brigham and Women's Hospital's Division of General Internal Medicine and Primary Care in Boston as a clinician researcher in the area of patient safety and medical informatics and associate director of the Brigham Center for Patient Safety Research and Practice. He is also an associate professor of Medicine at Harvard Medical School. He's won numerous honors for his work in patient safety, and in 2006 he was selected by *Modern Healthcare* as one of the "30 People for the Future"– national leaders most "likely to continue to shape health care in the years and decades ahead."

Gordy would take extraordinary means to make sure his patients got the right care. Like many of the med trainees, he was exemplary in his devotion to these people and would on occasion give them money to pay car fare. His concerns extended beyond medical concerns. Like me he believed medical care went beyond strictly technical approaches. The patient needed to enter a healthy environment when he left the hospital.

Since 1976, Mardge has worked at County, where she began her internal medical residency after attending Rush Medical College (where she and other students helped organize protests against the segregation of black and white obstetric patients leading to the successful integration of obstetric services at Rush at the late date of 1974).

In 1988 at County, Mardge started the Women and Children HIV Program to provide comprehensive medical and psychosocial services to women, their partners, and children, the first program of its kind in the nation. She was exceptional in her zeal, working very hard to treat women who were infected with and at that time dying of AIDS in unprecedented ways. She argued persuasively that they didn't just need doctors or pills (which early on did relatively little), but social workers, day care so they could attend their clinic visits, legal services to get the benefits to which they were entitled, substance use counselors and psychologists to address drug use and violence.

Mardge went on to become the director of Women's HIV Research at the CORE Center. Founded by the Cook County Bureau of Health Services and Rush-Presbyterian-St. Luke's Medical Center, CORE Center provides a comprehensive range of outpatient care to individuals and families affected by HIV & AIDS and other infectious diseases.

She has not confined her efforts to Chicago. Since 2004, Mardge has worked in Rwanda to facilitate HIV primary care for over 2000, women who were infected after being raped during the1994 genocide period.

Credit for creating and making the Committee to Save Cook County Hospital a powerful force goes to Linda, Gordy, Mardge, and other like-minded doctors and community leaders, including community activists Grace Leaming, Lon Berkeley and other house staff including, Jack Raba, Ron Sable, Arthur Hoffman, Bob Schiff, Ron Shansky, and Lambert King. This effort was essential. County was in grave financial trouble, yet its responsibilities continued to grow. Thus, the house staff, the community and I felt the least we could do was to fight for adequate resources.

Spoiler Alert: the hospital is still open for business as I write this some thirty-seven years later. But there were many days in the late 1970s and 1980s when the institution was on life support and we didn't know if it was going to make it. Come to think of it, that's still the case with County and other public hospitals far too often. At the same time County was in jeopardy in the '70s, Philadelphia closed its public hospital.

The argument for keeping County not only alive, but well, became increasingly necessary in 1979 when cries for closure intensified. Early that year, County Board Commissioner Joseph Tecson opined that private hospitals in Chicago had enough empty beds to take care of our entire patient population. He argued that these hospitals could be enticed to accept these patients if promised guaranteed payments.

One of the Committee's many organizing newsletters, dated October 30, 1979, addressed Tecson and other doomsdayers and privatizers. The document began with two questions. "Why is Cook County Hospital needed? Can the private hospitals take over if it closes?" The answer:

"Cook County Hospital is one of the largest public hospitals in the United States. It serves over 700,000 residents each year. The hospital has 1,453 beds and its Emergency Room has over 300,000 visits annually (the next largest E.R. in the city has only 100,000). Its outpatient visits have exceeded 300,000 in recent years. And its seven new satellite clinics are now providing 80,000 visitors annually with vital preventive and primary care. The fact that people regularly travel great distances from all across the county to come to the hospital is a strong indication of the need for and acceptance of its services.

There is no other facility that consistently guarantees health care regardless of ability to pay. Many private hospitals refuse to take Medicaid patients at all, and others impose quotas on the number they will see. In addition, Medicaid eligibility limits are so low in Illinois that any individual who makes over $1,800 annually and any family of four that makes over $4,200 cannot qualify for any medical benefits. County is the only hospital to which the increasingly large segment of our population—the working poor who do not have insurance—can turn for medical care.

Finally, the private sector has not shown any willingness to assume the immense task that CCH has shouldered. The deans of Chicago medical schools as well as the Chicago Hospital Council have indicated that their institutions are unable to take CCH's patients in the event that the hospital should be forced to reduce services. Moreover, a recent CCH inquiry of the Chicago area hospitals as to how many patients they could accept in the event that emergency transfers become necessary garnered only 134 available beds—only a fraction of which are capable of intensive care."

Other hospitals often stated that they were sending patients to County because they didn't have enough beds, had no vacancies. Maybe that was true on occasion. But more often than not—beds or no beds— those hospitals used County as a dumping ground for patients without private insurance or Medicaid.

At the same time, these hospitals saw another reason to send patients –many of whom did have insurance—to us. The fact was that some of our units offered the best care in the area for certain trauma and illness.

Those looking for a well-written chronicle of the effort to save the hospital during this period should turn to *County*, a book written by another doctor whom I am proud to call a "legacy," David Ansell. David, who came to the hospital in 1978, does an excellent job of explaining how County circa the 1970s was often ill-served by two competing public bodies charged with keeping it healthy—the governing commission and the Cook County Board. As I noted earlier, the board had been forced to cede governance, including jobs, to the commission in 1969—a healthy de-politici-zation. But the board had retained financial control. Such bifurca-tion of power and responsibility inevitably led to clashes—some in which the parties had the best of intentions, others in which selfishness trumped altruism.

This was our problem: County was running at a deficit. That tends to happen when most of your customers can't pay for the services you provide. It's not a viable business model, but then County wasn't a business. The shortfall had to be made up with increased revenue and/or service cutbacks—a situation that sounds eerily like the situation in the U.S. and around the world as I write this.

The same 1979 Committee to Save CCH newsletter that ex-plained why Cook County was needed also explained the finan-cial crisis. For example, in fiscal year 1978 there was a net loss of $40.4 million because the costs of inpatient operations and am-bulatory services far exceeded reimbursement. This, of course, resulted in a shortage of day-to-day revenues, resulting in among other things, "skip a check" paydays (or non-paydays!).

Missed paydays as a result of shortfalls didn't compare to unnecessary deaths. Ansell recalls the day power went out, caus-ing several ventilators to fail. Because there were no back-up gen-erators, two patients died.

What accounted for the annual deficit? The newsletter con-tinued: "The long-term crisis has resulted from the erosion of the financial bases for CCH along with the continued obligation to provide quality medical care for the sick, regardless of their abil-ity to pay."

The largest deficit came from the self-paying patients ("a euphemism referring to persons who have no form of third par-ty sponsorship such as Medicaid, Medicare, welfare or personal health insurance"). These self-payers comprised "the working poor, whom Medicaid was designated to help but whose income has been pushed by inflation above the Medicaid standard of $4,200 annually for a family of four." Indeed Medicaid, which had accounted for 63 percent of incoming payments in 1973, accounted for only 29 percent of such payments six years later. A public hospital is hard-pressed to operate under such circumstances.

The state could have helped ease the crisis by offering supplemental increases in Medicaid to account for the double-digit inflation of the late 1970s. But it didn't. At the same time, the county could have helped by forwarding $12 million in tax levies promised to the hospital. It didn't either.

Ignoring the fact that the crisis at County was the result of providing services without reimbursement, many critics cited waste and mismanagement as the prime reason for our woes. Inefficiency was no stranger to County. Nor were misplaced priorities and poor labor relations with the governing commission.

Truth be told, however, since the advent of the governing commission, the hospital had improved in most major respects. Under the County Board, loss of accreditation had been a real possibility. But after the commission had taken over, County had gone, as the handout noted, "from having a questionable reputation for patient care to gaining increasing respect in the community it serves. And it has gone from having serious staff deficiencies to having a highly regarded training program that attracts house staff from the country's major medical schools."

I don't mean to sound two-faced about the governing commission, with which I certainly had complaints and run-ins. But my objections were not with the concept of the commission. Rather, I did not like the way the commission exercised its power or, more accurately, abdicated its power to the director. I also thought the selectors could find more committed, less political commissioners who better reflected the demographics of our patients. In short, I wanted to see certain commissioners eliminated and replaced, not the commission.

Others disagreed. *Return the hospital to the control of the*

County Board which will then hire a private firm to manage the hospital, they said. *No,* replied our committee. There was no evidence to suggest a private management firm would have any better approach. Moreover, such a firm would still be faced with an underfinanced hospital. "Hospital management firms operate with a private sector mentality... Their emphasis is on profitability rather than community service." We cited a recent California study that concluded that the principal "innovative" move made by such firms upon taking over was to reduce personnel, the largest line-item of any hospital budget.

So what did the Committee to Save Cook County Hospital propose? Our approach was to deal with the issues of governance and finance. With respect to governance we urged a more professional, responsive commission with a representative constituency, a revised selection process to increase public involvement, greater input from the hospital work force, and legal certification of the relationship between commission and the county board.

None of this would matter if the financial ship couldn't be righted. Here we had a specific five-point plan:

1. An immediate infusion of funds to meet the remaining 1979 fiscal year payroll and expenses. Such money would come from the county and the state.

2. A long-term provision of a direct state subsidy to public hospitals on the basis of 50 percent matching funds for city and county contributions.

3. Changes in the Medicaid certification procedures and eligibility standards raised to at least the federal poverty level of $6,700.

4. Reforms by the Illinois Department of Public Aid.

5. Capital funding to construct a new Cook County Hospital.

We were realistic. "Obviously, the needs of Cook County Hospital cannot exist outside the financial limits of the responsible governmental bodies. However, we do not accept the contention that the health needs of working and poor people can only be met by increasing the taxes on working and poor people." Businesses should be taxed before the poor.

Because a public hospital is public it exists at the pleasure of the governmental bodies that fund it and the people who elect the representative bodies. The five-point plan recognized that the state legislature, the governor and his departments, the County Board and its president, and the City of Chicago were necessary players in the battle to save the hospital. Legislation was needed for funding and other changes.

A look through my files from this period reminds me of the intense effort we made to win the hearts and minds of numerous constituencies: elected and appointed officials, community leaders and the community in general, our patients, staff, and the media. To do so we sent letters, handed out leaflets and newsletters like the one described above, lobbied politicians, attended public hearings, and staged protests at Daley Plaza and elsewhere. Ansell's book reminds me that a silkscreen press was set up in the house staff offices to print posters that read: "Keep County Open. Health Care for People. Not Profit."

It's no secret that I have been a part of quite a few movements for change—some as a leader, some as a follower; some public, some behind the scenes. And some successful and some not so successful. I'm often asked what makes for a good fight in the name of a good cause. So for better or worse, here is Dr. Young's prescription for organizing an effective movement:

"Don't be afraid to say the same thing over and over again to lots of different audiences. They won't know that you have said it before, and those you have spoken to already might not remember and need to be reminded.

Always use sarcasm and humor.

Draw on every literary and artistic devise you can from Shakespeare to the Smothers Brothers.

Always connect lots of different struggles: from struggles against racism to struggles to end the war to struggles to get resources for the community.

Always remember to draw on and recall past great heroes,

171

such as Dr. King.

Don't be afraid to take on established offices of power, to struggle against them and make them become enabling resources for the movement. Yes, there are great risks to selling out, like becoming the boss at County, but in this there is also opportunity to inspire and catalyze and gain support for the struggle from below.

Know when to move on. My friends in the Committee to Save CCH and at County were disappointed when I left after a decade to form the Health & Medicine Policy Research Group (more on that later). Sometimes you need to strike a balance between long-term commitments— which are lifelong—and tactical strategies—which have to be constantly rethought.

Don't be afraid of being labeled a radical or socialist. Better to honestly state what your views are so no one can claim you are hiding anything and proudly wear your beliefs publicly. This has defanged many a redbaiter or right-winger."

How successful was our effort to save the hospital? I suppose you could proclaim it a winner because the old hospital stayed open and eventually a new hospital was built— which was one of our central demands—to replace the decrepit 1912 main hospital building. That, however, would be a sugar-coated assessment. For while we did garner considerable grassroots and media support for our effort, we took a punch in the gut in November 1979, just after offering that five-point plan. That's when the Illinois General Assembly killed the governing commission and returned control of the hospital to the Cook County Board. In the wake of this, Haughton resigned effective December 1.

The commission had been on thin ice for some time given the hospital's financial and labor woes. Whatever political capital it had built up evaporated when the commissioners bravely refused to slash services despite running out of money for the fiscal year. The state would eventually pony up money, but in return the commission had to go.

Even the Chicago *Tribune* editorial in the wake of this development said, "County deserves to live." It correctly noted that Governor James Thompson, County Board President George

Dunne and Chicago Mayor Jane Byrne expressed support for the hospital. The newspaper acknowledged that it was better to let the commission die instead of the hospital, but it also noted wisely that killing the commission was "not good. It remains to be shown that anyone else can run the operation with no more revenue than the Governing Commission had."

This all begs the question why would Dunne and the County Board want such a headache. The *Tribune* said what we all knew: "Some suspect the commissioners are expecting something in return for resumption of responsibility for a difficult operation. Are they drooling at the thought of thousands of patronage jobs?"

Although County was still alive as 1979 came to a close, the effort to save it was not over. The same problems would now be handled by a new body, albeit one that would have more state funds than its predecessor. But as 1980 unfolded little changed. A committee summary of 1980 noted several unwelcome developments:

- In May, the County Board engaged Hyatt Medical Management to run the hospital. Monthly fee: $200,000. "Beyond failing to resolve patient care problems, Hyatt's 'Financial Master Plan' threatens more serious consequences, including placement of cash registers in the Emergency Room and the demanding of cash deposits upon admission to the hospital."

- County Board President Dunne refused to renew the contracts of every labor union at the hospital. "This provocative action threatens the security and working conditions of all employees, contributing to lower morale and harming recruitment attempts."

- On the positive side, in February 1980, the County had doubled its support for the hospital. This had prevented a repetition of the crisis faced in the fall of 1979. "However, by delays in orders and failing to fill the hundreds of vacant positions, the County Board is still starving the hospital financially."

- "The dismantling of the community clinic system established under the governing commission constitutes a serious setback for care to Chicago's many underserved areas."

While these developments didn't necessarily threaten County's survival, the hospital's future remained up in the air thanks to our West Side neighbor, Rush Presbyterian St. Luke's Medical Center. For several years, the relationship between County and this private hospital had been contentious. Matters had come to a head in 1978, when the Rush erected a wall on Paulina Street, blocking the major route to Cook County and University of Illinois Hospitals' Emergency Rooms. This brazen blockade which threatened the well-being of our patients led to mass protests by our staff and the community.

The already tense situation was exacerbated in March of 1980 by the Rush's president, James Campbell. He had long argued for a reorganization of health care services, teaching, and research in the Chicago metropolitan area. Now he offered a plan titled "Rationalizing the Health Care System in Chicago." The "Campbell Plan" proposed organizing the Chicago area into five to seven "comprehensive integrated care and education networks." Each network would be headed by an academic health center.

The Committee to Save Cook County Hospital called for action to defeat the plan, noting that the networks would eliminate community say in health planning because all power would be vested in the academic centers. As these centers were focused on teaching and research, primary care would take a backseat. Moreover, the plan incentivized private hospitals to "close the public hospital and keep it closed at the first sign of a worker strike or other 'disruption.'" Campbell proposed using public funds to support his plan. This constituted "another blow at the public sector and the population it serves."

A Committee handout quoted Dr. Vicente Navarro of Johns Hopkins. Saying he was "profoundly distressed," Dr. Navarro explained, "(It) seems to have been drafted without any formal participation from public authorities, consumer representatives, community organizations, labor unions, etc... It is a blueprint aimed at a complete fiasco."

County survived the Campbell Plan just as it survived the misguided efforts of the Haughtons, Dunnes, and Tecsons of the world. I survived, too. But by the middle of 1980, I decided that it was time to move on.

(A footnote: In this You Tube age, it is possible to get an idea of what County and its environs looked like in 1979. That year a BBC film crew took up residency in the hospital to produce that documentary, "I CALL IT MURDER," which aired in the UK and can still be seen on the Internet at http://vimeo.com/22358840)

After the documentary aired, I received scores of well-written letters from Great Britain from a self-identified cross-class base. The letters praised the hospital and its staff (which was perceived, romantically, as having pitted good vs. evil) against a heartless, racist white power structure. Moreover, in addition to sending their prayers and blessings, the correspondents enclosed pound notes, checks, and offers to come work at the hospital.

Some of the writers were a bit smug about the socialized medicine that they enjoy in comparison to the U.S. system of health care. A whiff of condescension was evident in the film itself, as an Irish doctor working at County professed amazement at our way of doing business.

The production captured the reality of the hospital, but perhaps inevitably stressed the more dramatic, violent, and medically intriguing aspects of the institution. In the process, unwittingly I'm sure, the filmmakers created a picture that would have been politically disastrous if shown in Chicago.

Viewers saw a predominantly white professional staff (an inaccurate chance result of the particular scenes broadcast, since we had a very large minority professional contingent) treating an undeserving black lumpen. The film showed poignant examples of the most alienated of our patients: a heroin-addicted prostitute chatting with an atypically sympathetic police officer, a passive-aggressive teenaged hemophiliac berating the staff for alleged bad care, and a bloody scene of a black middle-aged couple who inflicted violence on one another.

To its credit the film also showed helpless souls shipped to County after being denied treatment at the hospitals they had rushed to after being attacked or falling ill. Neither the patients nor the staff believed those private hospitals' explanations that they didn't have beds. Clearly they had been denied treatment because they didn't have insurance, Medicaid, or the means to pay.

In perhaps the most poignant scene, an older gentleman on a hospital bed pulls money out from his wallet and attempts to pay a nurse for the care he is receiving. The nurse repeatedly tells the patient, "This is County, you don't have to pay."

I relished scenes like that, but was glad the documentary wasn't shown in Chicago, as the scenes could definitely have been exploited by local bigots to seek even further funding cuts.

Mardge Cohen and Gordy Schiff

After over 31 years at Cook County Hospital, Mardge and Gordy moved to Boston. Gordy is currently Associate Director of the Center for Patient Safety Research and Practice and Associate Professor of Medicine at Harvard Medical School. Mardge practices at Boston Health Care for the Homeless Program, continues research on women with HIV in Chicago, and is medical director of Women's Equity in Access to Care and Treatment (WE-ACTx) in Rwanda. Gordy and Mardge are members of PNHP. Both are self-confessed "serial boundary crossers" crossing boundaries to help and reach out to their patients, behaviors they learned from Quentin Young.

We trained with Quentin Young as young doctors in internal medicine at Cook County in the 1970's and have been lucky to work with him on dozens on occasions since. Quentin was our teacher and mentor. Quentin reminds us of a cartoon where there are two people in front of a firing squad in blindfolds, about to be executed. One turns to the other and says, "I have a plan!" That is Quentin and he has brought us in front of many firing squads throughout our time together: public hearings, all night vigils, bus trips to Springfield, historical foundings of new organizations and press conferences where there is no press.

Quentin showed us the idea of having power by sharing information. Instead of hoarding information, Quentin was the opposite of that due to some combination of his ego, where he had to tell everybody everything, his democratic impulses and his strategic understanding of how information is power. He embodied his favorite quote of Frederick Douglass, "Knowledge makes a man unfit to be a slave." Another illustration of something profoundly influential that Quentin taught us was speaking truth to power. He didn't shrink away, never hid his politics and never compromised his ideas. At County, we would converge at his office at the end of the day, yell at him and he would tell us what happened and why. That message of open communication resonated with us at County and that style of dealing with people is now widespread throughout this city because of Quentin.

Quentin's relationship with his patients knew no boundaries. Organizing for political demonstrations, lobbying politicians, disrupting visits for key phone calls and meeting outside of the office, were all part of how he appreciated and served patients. Ultimately, Quentin believed that doctors and patients have to work together saying, "the personalization of the individual and destruction of the community, the emblems of our time, are conspicuously manifested in the role models enacted in healthcare settings. A revised concept would envision changes in the roles of the physicians, nurses and other health providers and in the role of the patient who would come to be regarded as the keeper of his or her own medical health, capable of intelligent decisions when he or she became ill." It's that alliance that will change the health system so it is accessible, universal and designed around meeting the needs of people and not profits.

One last thing we learned from Quentin was how to use medicine as a metaphor and how to diagnose some of the problems with the health system. He wrote that "Medical Savings Accounts are the latest scam on American patients and taxpayers. They're based on the incorrect assumption that Americans are addicts for health care and that if there isn't a dollar barrier, they'll overconsume. In fact, Americans get fewer doctors' visits than people in countries with universal health care." Quentin is always prescribing this or that.

Some of the wisdom he provided was through simple and famous Quentin lines including; "Patients are not gluttonous addicts, eager to rush to the doctor to have needles stuck into them or tubes stuck down their throats or rectums." "Constipated legislative processes in Springfield." "Some of these incremental health reforms that are being proposed will do as much good as a couple of aspirins will do for a brain tumor. We have to make a diagnosis and give treatment. The diagnosis is clear, we have a failed experiment with market forces."

He always found time for us and everyone else, which is a model for us and we strive to be mentors for others. We would call him when we needed input into key professional, personal and political decisions. He listened, got it immediately and helped tremendously. From his witty and prescient metaphors to his lessons in talking truth to power and information sharing to his commitment to a doctor-patient partnership, Quentin taught/showed us what it really meant to listen, empower and partner with patients to make them better and to make a better world.

Twelve

On July 16, 1980, I sent a handwritten letter to Rowine Brown, the Medical Director of Cook County Hospital. It read in part:

> *Dear Dr. Brown,*
> *I regret to inform you, with this letter, of my resignation, as chairman of the Department of Medicine effective January 15, 1981... I want to express gratitude for the opportunity to work at this vital institution serving the poor. My every wish is for its future good fortune.*

In a statement expanding upon the letter, I noted that, "Given the fact that I fought for my job in federal court when I was fired on two different occasions, it cannot be reasonably suggested that I do not value the position or would give it up lightly."

So why go? "I have decided to resign because a series of developments have convinced me that unless there is new support and remedy of these situations, it would not be possible for this wonderful and historic institution to continue its mission, offering health care to the hundreds of thousands of sick poor in this area who depend on it."

The six developments that I cited were the usual suspects: funding, unreasonable patient charges, the maturing of plans by private sector powers to further destabilize and divide up the hospital (such as the Campbell Plan), denial of the benefits of unionization to the CCH work force, mismanagement by the Hyatt Hospital Management Association, and the problems with the County's Jail Health Service.

While the first five developments were discussed in the previous chapter, I have not yet explained the situation with respect to the jail. I was and remain proud that between 1973 and 1976, the Department of Medicine dramatically improved the health services for the 5,000 inmates in the County Jail (over the course of a year 50,000 inmates entered the institution). But in 1978 Cermak Hospital, the on-site medical institution for the jail, had been closed. The closure was understandable; it was a tiny, tiny facility within four miles of CCH and it was becoming harder and harder to staff since Jim Haughton would not allow attending physicians to be there. It had outgrown its role as an inpatient facility providing complex care and surgeries that could be more adequately provided at the nearby Cook County Hospital. The result was that all hospitalized medical and psychiatric patients were now brought to a special prison ward on the 7th floor of the A building (ward 75 locked unit) at County. This further depleted jail services.

Problems abounded. In 1976, Haughton had placed Vivian Sodini as the administrator of the jail. This resulted in the departure of the able medical director, Bert King. More dysfunction: we had given management a proposal to integrate services at the jail with our resources at CCH so that we could have adequate back up for the residents, but had not received a satisfactory response. Haughton basically told the residents they weren't needed anymore and sent them back to the hospital. He brought in private doctors who were not trained in correctional health.

My vision for what this health system could be was crumbling. By 1979 we heard that the County was paying more in legal consultation to cover malpractice lawsuits against the jail health service than it was paying for health care at the jail. Tragic.

(When the medical director position opened up at the jail, I encouraged my friend and former resident, Jack Raba, to take the job. He refused several times. He finally agreed to write up a list of demands and conditions under which he would take the position and present these to Haughton. Haughton agreed, and Jack took leadership. I am very proud of the fact that the next generation of physician correctional health leaders across the U.S. largely came out of the program I created—-Jack, Ron Shansky, Mike Puisis,

Bobby Cohen, and Bert King to name a few.)

By now I trust you have figured out that I don't shy away from a battle. Some –including colleagues, friends, and family— may even say I relish a good fight. So again: why leave an institution I loved instead of staying to fight from the inside where I might have some clout—no matter how small? I explained to the press: "I stepped down to call attention to the areas of malignant neglect, convinced that only a public examination of the issues offered hope of remedy."

So what have I learned over the years about when it is right to stay and fight from within, and when it's right to quit to make a point and then fight from the outside? The answer to this question is two other questions: How can you best effect a change, and how important is the issue? County Hospital meant the world to me. But my personal experience and reflections told me I could now do more from the outside by agitating and organizing for change than I could if I continued on the inside.

In announcing my resignation, I also said: "At the present time I am going to no other institution nor am I leaving for a different attractive medical situation." Since I'd given six months, not two weeks, notice, I had time to figure out my next move. One obvious option was to return to my private medical practice. Doing so would not preclude involvement in some other public activity to improve the delivery of health services to the needy. But what kind of activity?

Enter my long-time friend, John McKnight. I had first met John when he was at the Chicago Commission for Human Relations in the 1950s and he joined our group, The Committee to End Discrimination in Chicago Medical Institutions. We developed a close friendship which has lasted to today. One of the things I most admired about John was his ability to see what might be possible in dealing with society's most complicated problems. He saw opportunities for change that nobody else might envision. He was, therefore, the most logical person to consult when I was facing the possibility of a seismic shift in my career.

A little background on John: After graduating from Northwestern University and serving in the Navy, he returned to Chicago and began working for several activist organizations, including the Chicago Commission for Human Relations, the first municipal civil rights agency. There he learned the Saul Alinsky trade called *community organizing*. This was followed by the directorship of the Illinois American Civil Liberties Union, where he organized local chapters throughout the state.

When John Kennedy was elected president, John was recruited into the federal government, where he worked with a new agency that created the affirmative action program. Later, he was appointed the Midwest director of the United States Commission on Civil Rights, where he worked with local civil rights and neighborhood organizations.

In 1969, John's alma mater, Northwestern University, invited him to return and help initiate a new department called the Center for Urban Affairs. This was a group of interdisciplinary faculty doing research designed to support urban change agents and progressive urban policy. The appointment was an act of courage on the part of the university. It gave John a tenured professorship, though he had only a bachelor's degree.

While at the center and its successor, the Institute for Policy Research, John and a few of his colleagues focused their research on urban neighborhoods. The best-known result of this work was the formulation of an understanding of neighborhoods based on the utility of local resources, capacities, and relationships. This work was documented in a guide titled, *Building Communities from the Inside Out*. It described an approach to community building that became a major development strategy practiced across the world. During this time John was one of the trainers of a young community organizer named Barack Obama.

With a resume like the above, it's obvious why I turned to John after I made the decision to leave County and needed counsel to explore the next phase. And of course he didn't disappoint. His quick reply, as if he'd been thinking of little else, was that I should form a progressive health policy think tank, with a working board and small staff, independent of any institutional ties and focused on local health policy issues. In a time of diminished federal funding for health care, this "action tank"—free of institutional fetters in order to preserve program integrity—would operate as a humble, grassroots organization despite an ambitious agenda

How does an idea for a grassroots action tank turn into a reality? Here's what happened after John and I had our first discussion. The two of us decided to call together activists who we knew were committed to health care as a right and who knew that there were obstacles, organic and functional, to that concept. The original group (including Lon Berkeley, Iris Blustain, Doug Cassel, Jack Connelly, Effie Ellis, Sybille Fritzsche, Mike Gelder, Don Goldhammer, Yolanda Hall, Jenny Knauss, Grace Leaming, Carron Maxwell, Nancy Mikelsons, Ron Shansky, Pat Terrell, as well as John and myself) was eclectic, but represented health activists John and I had known and worked with over the previous decade.

We met in various living rooms for several months as we plodded along trying to define the organization. We were certain that the concepts of health and medicine were not synonymous. We wanted to deal with the contradictions in these words and what they meant. The synthesis of Health and Medicine Policy Research Group (HMPRG) as it was finally named, was that it would be independent of any institution, that we would oppose the exploiters of the health system—specifically corporations—and that the board would be a working board, not a membership one. In fact we were quite elitist; we wanted the board and small staff to be the determinants of what we did. For example, we hired Pat Terrell as our first executive director, half time at the grand salary of $50/week.

What we were trying to do—influence the health system in Chicago and Illinois—was ambitious and maybe a bit naïve, but thanks to the virtue of our cause, it's remarkable what a small group of unequivocally committed people have been able to accomplish over these thirty-two years. We could not have imagined back then that we would now have a board of over thirty people, a budget of over $1 million and a staff of a dozen continuing to act on the principles we were founded upon.

While the original group was composed of Young and McKnight friends and colleagues, we all struggled with the decision of whom else to invite to join us. Although we didn't formally use our later-established policy of a "single veto," there was definitely an effort to seek a consensus on recommended people, enlist like-minded activists whom someone in the group knew and who brought some diversity to the mix of current members.

One important element in starting an organization is selecting its name. Let it be known that I am never part of an organization with fewer than six words in its title, and I've been part of a lot of organizations. We cared most about the conflict between health and medicine and the tension between these concepts has been instructive to us always.

Initially we were going to call our new organization Chicago Health Advocacy Research Group, or, cleverly, CHARG. But we decided against that name, in part because we weren't certain we would only focus on Chicago; what we were seeking was universal, even if we were only focusing on Chicago and Illinois. Eventually we decided to call ourselves the Health Policy, Education and Research Group (HPERG). However, soon thereafter, we had changed that to Health and Medicine Policy Research Group.

In my files I've found the draft of a document that offered the public an introduction to the organization. Dated June 30, 1981, the document explains that we were a not-for-profit charitable trust formed "to respond to the crises in the existing health care system." Those crises? "Government leaders no longer view health care as one of the most important responsibilities of government. Rather, government spending for health care is labeled one of the major causes of our diseased economy."

Beyond this, "The public no longer takes pride in the achievements in health. Rather, malpractice, over-utilization and tragic stories of waste and neglect in our institutions command our attention."

There were three different dimensions to the crisis of the day: economic, political, and systemic. The national health bill in 1980 was $250 million, nearly ten percent of the country's gross national product. We estimated that dollar figure would triple by 1990, with health care consuming 25 percent of the GDP. (For your information: $2.7 trillion was spent on health care in the U.S.

in 2012.) "Yet with so much of the national fortune expended on health care, the U.S. health measures have not improved dramatically over the past twenty years. (Many other) countries now score better than the U.S. in life expectancy, infant mortality, and days lost from school and work."

The newly installed Reagan Administration seemed to have little interest in addressing these problems. Our document stated: "The nation no longer has a goal to improve its health and especially the health of its minorities and disadvantaged....National and local leaders make decisions which kill or slowly strangle the only agencies—public health departments, community health centers, public general hospitals—which have contributed to the achievements that have been made in life expectancy and infant mortality."

In their place, private academic medical centers and corporations dedicated to growth and profit now dominated the decision-making process. The environmental and occupational causes of disease and disability, not to mention the declining health services to our rapidly expanding County prison population, were being ignored.

What was our group going to do about this? "RESEARCH the major medical, political, and social determinants of illness... EDUCATE the public about the hazards inherent in the existing health care system... Analyze HEALTH POLICY decisions to identify and expose the corporate beneficiaries of the existing system." Such work would serve as "the foundation to advocate changes in the system..."

Our structure was important. We created four task forces, each one directed at a major cause of ill health. The task forces included: studying the health system as a whole; studying the impact of institutions, both within and outside the system; studying the impact of the environment and industry; and studying the health impact of public policy, specifically the diversion of tax dollars away from public programs which directly delivered services to those who needed them most.

Then what? We would "combine meticulous investigative research with public education, utilizing such forums as journals, conferences, press conferences and releases, media appearances, testimony at legislative and regulatory hearings, conferences and workshops, legal action, and academic curricula."

Pretty ambitious, to be sure, but, "(We) can achieve (our) objectives. Each of (our) 21 founders has a longstanding commitment to overcome the nation's health care problems. As educators, physicians, health planners, managers, system designers, government and institutional workers, mental health providers, union organizers, nutritionists, and attorneys," we offered a mix that was "essential to truly comprehend and analyze the existing system and advocate changes which will put it back on course."

Other helpful ingredients? Close relationships with educators and the media and our location. "Chicago has long been the nation's capital for health policy. Situated here are the national headquarters of the American Medical Association, American Hospital Association, Blue Cross/Blue Shield Association, Joint Commission on the Accreditation of Hospitals, American Dental Association, many professional organizations and medical specialty societies, several giant pharmaceutical complexes, five academic medical centers."

I was named chairman and president, and continued to have both those titles until the early 1990s, when we were beginning to grow and realized we needed more administrative and financial oversight—not my strengths. At that point we decided that I would be chairman (the title I retain to this day) and the group would decide upon a president. Incidentally, the board could, according to our bylaws, vote me out as chairman at any time. So far they have not chosen to do so.

Before 1981 had ended, we were already making waves. "Innovative answer to the Medicaid mess," cried a Chicago *Sun-Times* editorial. "A new public interest organization, the Health and Medicine Policy Research Group, suggests restructuring Medicaid in a way that can appeal to clients, health care providers, officials and taxpayers alike—while coping with the decades' shrinking budgetary expenditures."

Citing several demonstration projects, we were advocating shifting responsibility for the poor from the state to county governments, which historically had shouldered responsibility for public health. Under our plan the state legislature would establish an Illinois Health Service Authority empowered to distribute Medicaid funds to the counties on a per capita basis and then monitor the results.

I should note that in our early days, there was some outside tension from activists who felt that HMPRG was draining energy that might otherwise be focused on the Committee to Save Cook County Hospital. As time went on I think we all grew to realize that more people meant more energy. Ultimately I think the focus of the Committee to Save CCH got incorporated into the work of HMPRG.

Sometimes we met weekly, sometimes bi-weekly or less frequently depending on the urgency of the problem we were addressing. Our first office was in the heart of downtown Chicago and it was a sub-lease from an organization led by one of our board members. Other local community and health groups were called upon for advice and expertise, thereby promoting the sharing of resources.

The board and staff chose projects to work on based on perceived community need and urgency, our skills and the skills of people we knew we could call upon, and our interests. All board members were committed to working with staff on projects. In fact one of our early guidelines was that at least two board members must be committed to working on a project/issue before it was accepted as a priority.

Public education was achieved through all available public forums: professional and popular publications, press briefings, radio and television, legislative and other public hearings, conferences, workshops, academic curricula, legal action and our journal *Health & Medicine* (in which we published our work three times each year from 1982 to1987). The journal was to be a distillation of our group's work, a communication with our friends around the country about creative efforts to change the way that health care is perceived and delivered. We were committed to making the magazine a forum for dialog and debate that could be of value to those working to guarantee all people a health system that is effective and equitable. Ultimately the journal was too expensive for us to sustain, but I remain proud of what we wrote about and the thousands of people who we reached through it.

Some of the first projects we worked on included:

Medicaid Reform:

Medicaid cutbacks in the early 1980s under the Reagan administration led our Public Policy Task Force to think about and propose to the state a new way to organize the Medicaid program. As the *Sun Times* reported, this would be achieved by giving the counties authority to organize the program to reflect the clients' needs rather than the appetites of the corporate medical industry. Although our decentralization proposal was not implemented, it was debated in our state legislature and proposed as legislation.

We also launched the Citizens Coalition for Medicaid Reform, which wielded significant influence by increasing meaningful client participation in Medicaid and redirecting some of the Medicaid budget toward local services and programs. HMPRG continues to work on Medicaid reform to this day, joining with partners in government, advocacy, research and provider groups to ensure that Medicaid services are comprehensive and accessible.

Occupational Health History:

To build on the important relationship between work and health, HMPRG joined with local unions, the Chicago Area Committee on Occupational Safety and Health, the Occupational Medicine Department at Cook County Hospital, and the Suburban Health Systems Agency to develop a new approach to the use of a personal work history form. This project, funded by the Illinois Division of the American Cancer Society, demonstrated HMPRG's unique approach to addressing issues, while at the same time making connections with other groups I had previously helped foster like CACOSH and CCH's Occupational Medicine Department.

With key staff support from Leslie Nickels, this personal

work history form was designed to encourage workers to consider and record health-related factors where they work. Then, by encouraging them to voluntarily share this document with their personal physician and their unions, it would not only help improve the diagnosis and treatment of occupational diseases by physicians, but also enable unions to identify suspicious trends in the workplace. This was a win-win-win for patient empowerment, organizing, and health care outcomes.

Reducing Infant Mortality:

Wanting to launch a coalition focused on addressing infant mortality in Chicago, HMPRG began, as it frequently found effective to do, with a conference. Community members spoke loudly against the health care and political institutions which were responsible for inadequate maternal and infant care. This was followed by workshops focusing on advocacy strategies to address these challenges. Over 400 people attended the conference and during the media build-up to the conference, Chicago's Mayor Jane Byrne announced a $1.2 million dollar program to tackle infant mortality—the timing was not a coincidence.

Through the conference HMPRG launched the Healthy Mothers and Babies Coalition—initially about seventy organizations and individuals. We hired a staff person for the coalition and eventually, as has become our hallmark, the coalition was launched into its own organization and still thrives today, under a different name.

It's worth noting that we had no money to hold this conference, but we recklessly went ahead with it because we knew how important the issues were. We arrived at the office on the Monday after the conference to find a check for $10,000 from one of the insurance companies we had asked for support. Were we lucky!!

Study Tours of Urban Health Systems:

We led study tours—which we called urban Public Health Care System Study Tours— in the US and Canada with legislators, civic and community leaders. Our purpose was to showcase the ways in which Canada and other US cities had organized health services and how they might be models for us to follow.

Cook County Hospital:
We convened a task force to formulate a position on the future of Cook County Hospital that envisioned a new centralized hospital with community-based, integrated out-patient facilities across the county. Eventually our vision was realized (see previous chapters and below), although budget challenges continue to threaten the viability of the system to this day.

Since that earliest effort more than thirty years ago, HMPRG has thought big and accomplished much, under the leadership of executive directors Pat Terrell, Linda Diamond Shapiro and a couple of others for short periods— and, since 1993, Margie Schaps, and a working board that really works.

Some examples of causes and issues that we have played major roles in over the last several years:

Securing a new Cook County Hospital and the independent board for the County Health System.
In the late 1990s I was appointed, along with many captains of industry and civic leaders (my friend Lester Crown comes to mind) to a commission charged with making recommendations to the County leadership on whether we should build a new Cook County Hospital and if so, how large it should be. We hired the financial consulting firm of Grant Thornton to do the financial projections and feasibility study.

The commission recommended a 450-bed inpatient facility. Most of us knew that was too small, but we also recognized it was the limit of what we could get. Nobody in the country was building new public hospitals at the time and this size was consistent with the size of large private hospitals being developed.

I did not just want a new building—I was fond of saying I did not have an edifice complex— I wanted to preserve the commitment to a broad range of specialty and community based services. After much blood, sweat, and tears, we won the day. We were finally on our way to building a hospital that would be efficient for the staff and deserving of the population we serve.

The hospital opened in 2003 . I know that while the struggles continue for this system and all public systems, the opening of this hospital and its existence as an institution that takes care of the most marginalized impoverished people in our community has been very important. Health & Medicine, the Committee to Save CCH, Ruth Rothstein, Pat Terrell and dozens of others have much to be proud of.

You've heard a lot about Mr. Haughton and the independent board of the 1970s, but once that was abolished, governance went back to the County Board. By the early 2000s, with the less-than-effective Todd Stroger as head of the County Board and Dr. Robert Simon as the CEO of the system, we knew we needed a new governance structure once again. I called upon my union friends at SEIU and AFSCME, Citizen Action, a host of community groups, and some brave County Commissioners (primarily Larry Suffredin) to write an ordinance that would create an independent board. We won, and in 2007 that board was established. It's not perfect, and we wish it had more authority, but it was a great step forward.

Passing legislation to establish freestanding birth centers (FSBCs) in Illinois:

This has been a long and very hard road in Illinois. Board member Lon Berkeley, who had become familiar while in Rhode Island with free-standing birth centers as a low cost, safe option for low risk women, wanted to bring this relatively new delivery model to Illinois. Teaming up with nurse-midwife Gina Novick, HMPRG convened in 1984 a task force to explore how to accomplish this.

To achieve our aims, we organized a statewide coalition of activists, physicians, midwives, other healthcare provider and community groups who understood the value of FSBCs to rural communities without services, to underserved communities where culturally and linguistically appropriate services didn't exist, and to all women who wanted and deserved choices in childbirth.

As HMPRG always does, we worked with many tools (such

as educating through conferences, using the media to tell stories of birth centers, and conducting research about birth centers in other states), and partnered with other supportive organizations. My role was to provide the medical voice when we needed a physician and to make connections to key state politicians with whom I had relationships. Finally, in 2007, thanks to the resilient leadership of Lon, and Gayle Riedmann, our nurse midwife board member, who took over leadership of the Birth Center Task Force in 1989, we were able to shift the position of the American College of Obstetrics and Gynecology, neutralize the Illinois State Medical Society and Illinois Hospital Association positions, and pass legislation paving the way for the regulations needed to establish birth centers in Illinois.

Multiple barriers had been placed before us. Opponents insinuated that abortions would be done in birth centers (not true), or that these would be "drive-by" births. But we were ultimately successful with the invaluable help of key staff in the state legislature and governor's office (including previous HMPRG board members Michael Gelder and Jerry Stermer, who were very familiar with this issue). This was quite a victory for us, and we expect that the first birth center in the state will open in early 2014.

Providing leadership and research that supports Illinois' movement toward a long-term care system focused on home- and community-based services

In 2001, at the urging of board members Martha Holstein and Michael Gelder, HMPRG decided to focus on the problem of how state Medicaid dollars were spent on older, frail adults in Illinois. Relative to many states, Illinois spent a disproportionate amount of these dollars on nursing home care relative to home and community based services. To us, this was wrong. Working again in coalition with others, we were able to pass a law establishing a state committee dedicated to rebalancing. Since then we've been successful in moving some money away from institutional care to home and community based care.

More recently, we've collaborated with hospitals and community providers to address the national challenge of hospital readmissions for older adults—difficult and often disorienting to the senior, and costly for the system. Under the leadership of board member Robyn Golden, we've developed the "Bridge Model," a social work-based model applicable on a nationwide base that supports seniors in transition from hospital to home and supports them to stay in their home—an improvement for the patient and their family and a cost savings for the system.

Addressing the problem of unmet health and mental health needs in prisons, particularly among the most marginalized youth

I and HMPRG had a long standing interest in improving health care to incarcerated people, so in 2003 we had a conference exploring the health needs of the most vulnerable prison populations. What we learned attuned us to the growing numbers of girls in the prisons and jails in Illinois and the revolving door system these kids seem to be in partly because their health and mental health issues are not addressed. As a result HMPRG organized a task force of like-minded groups and was successful in a campaign to hire a staff person in the Cook County Juvenile Temporary Detention Center focused on programming and services for girls. This was quite an accomplishment and I am very proud that we took this on.

More recently our attention has been on the growing population of LGBTQ youth in the court system. State and County leaders asked us for help in addressing staff training and services for this expanding demographic. We have now trained prison and jail staff across the state in the special needs of this population and have spearheaded the successful effort to enact a policy in Cook County about staff training regarding working with LGBTQ youth.

Creating opportunities for health professional students to focus their altruistic interests in communities of need

In 1994 I was invited to a meeting at the Chicago Community Trust (the largest community foundation in Chicago, which had been a consistent funder of HMPRG since the beginning) with leaders of Chicago's medical schools to talk about starting a Chicago "branch" of the Albert Schweitzer Fellowship—a program begun in Boston and housed at Harvard Medical School that provides exceptional graduate level health professional students (medical, nursing, social work, etc). an opportunity to design and implement projects to improve the health and well-being of underserved communities. The fellows often focus their efforts on addressing the social determinants of health, such as literacy, violence prevention, and promotion of healthy nutrition and healthy behaviors. The program is a unique opportunity of these like-minded, aspiring change agents from different schools and disciplines to work together to develop public symposia on health and social issues facing these populations. Boston was the mother-ship of the program. There were, however, three others in the country, and the folks out East were interested in starting a program in Chicago. I think I was invited to this meeting because I had run the Urban Preceptorship program at the University of Illinois in the '70s and had some experience in related activities. I was really interested in what I was hearing at the Trust meeting, but when it came time for someone, on behalf of some institution, to step up and say they would host the program in Chicago, I held back.

When I returned to the office and told Linda Shapiro and Margie Schaps, at the time our co-executive directors, that I did not offer HMPRG as the host, they replied: "Why not? We want those students."

I held back because they and others often accused me (correctly so) of never saying no! I thought they were going to applaud my self-control. Boy was I wrong. Soon HMPRG had a new program.

It turns out to have been a marvelous decision to host the Chicago expression of the Albert Schweitzer Fellowship. Since 1995, nearly 450 Chicago Schweitzer Fellows have completed over 90,000 hours of community service at more than 150 community-based sites. They meet monthly in our office to talk about the boulders they face in working with hard-to-reach populations, to learn about health policy, and to explore what working in interdisciplinary teams can mean to improving the lives of the poor. We see these fellows as the on-the-ground expression of much of our policy and research work. In 2006 we created the first-in-the-nation "Fellows for Life" program to help support former Schweitzer Fellows as they maintain their commitment to the underserved.

As you must know by now, I love teaching. I love spending time with bright young people who want to do good and who care about social justice. The Schweitzer program has given me endless opportunities over the last nineteen years to host these students at my house for meals, to give talks to them about health justice, and to support them in realizing their potential.

**

In addition to the dozens of projects HMPRG has taken on over the years—some won, some lost—we have earned a reputation as the leading local health policy center and have gained the respect of local, state and congressional elected officials. Local—and sometimes national—media turn to our staff, board, and me for comment, information, and referrals on a regular basis.

We've infiltrated the system! We have served or contributed to the health transition teams of elected officials, including Chicago mayors, Cook County board presidents, state legislators, governors, and congressional representatives, as well as orienting new public leaders at the state, county, and city levels. The governor, the Illinois Attorney General, the county board president and more have appointed our board and staff to serve on countless local and state commissions and have named several to leadership positions, from the Governor's Senior Health Policy Advisor (Michael Gelder), to the Executive Director of the Illinois Caucus for Adolescent Health (Jenny Knauss), to Executive Director of the Midwest Latino Health Research Center (Aida Giachello), to Executive Directors of local Federally Qualified Health Centers (Carmen Velasquez, Fred Rachman and others), to members of the Cook County Health and Hospitals System Independent Board of Directors (Heather O'Donnell), to Medical Director of the Cook County Health and Hospitals System (Claudia Fegan).

The life expectancy of most grassroots not-for-profits is considerably less than thirty years. How has HMPRG survived and thrived? First of all we fill a need. Independent and nimble, we are an essential source for the diverse constituency described above—media, legislators and other public officials, foundations, and other not for profits and ad hoc coalitions.

Just having the product is not enough. We have accomplished what we have by joining with others who share our vision. Policy change is hard and can only be done by building coalitions, conducting solid research, and articulating a clear vision to the media, policy makers and the public. I never expected this group to accomplish so much and to be a leader in so many spheres. But it has and I am proud that I have been the leader of such a robust action-think tank for these 32 years.

As for me, Health and Medicine has provided a wonderful venue to impact health policy on a local and state level and to marry my comittment to health justice and social justice movements in general. I recall one very cold winter morning in 2008 walking into the HMPRG office, and asking the question I asked every day "So what have we done this day to fight the forces of reaction?", to which I got the usual response from staff of all of the activities of the day thus far. Margie and I got to work on various projects. A couple of hours passed, and I put on my coat—"Where are you going? We have deadlines to meet", Margie said. To which I replied, "I have work to do, and you should do it with me. I'm going to join the Republic Window Workers marching at Bank of America." Republic Windows had closed its doors in violation of federal labor law that required companies to give workers 60 days notice. The workers were also being cheated out of more than $1.5 million in health care benefits, severance and vacation time. "There is nothing more important than standing with the workers." Margie put on her coat, and we marched with the workers. Our work could wait.

By no means are we done. Since this is my book, I will take this opportunity to note our ambitious agenda for the future:

- Strengthening the Chicago/Cook County and regional health care safety net
- Addressing the health needs of court involved youth
- Developing a coalition and advocate for a statewide single-payer health insurance system
- Building the Schweitzer Fellows for Life program to support all former Chicago area Schweitzer Fellows in their commitment to underserved
- Recommending new ways to improve health care quality for people with disabilities
- Promoting innovative models of care under the state's Medicaid reform plans
- Providing leadership to reform long-term care in Illinois and research and policy promotion to ensure older adults have economic security
- Assisting with the implementation of the Affordable Care Act's mission of improved quality better health care, improved outcomes, and reduced per capita cost—even though we believe the current law is inadequate
- Helping develop and train the health care workforce, including new providers (like community health workers), new models of caregiving (supporting family caregivers), and new systems of care (regional health systems)

The past thirty years has validated the importance of organizational independence—which allows HMPRG to respond to immediate threats and problems that arise even as we work on long term policy agendas. HMPRG has had the luxury to choose its causes based on what our board and staff see as demanding attention, and we have chosen well. I've seen HMPRG gain popular support and gain the respect of other health and medical groups. Even when they disagree with our policy formulation, they know the quality of our work is high.

As noted I have been Chairman since Day One. At first I was able to come to the office and work to amplify the staff capacity two days a week on a voluntary basis (I practiced medicine the other three days each week). As time passed I reduced my medical practice and spent first three, and then five days each week (since 2008) at the office, splitting my time between HMPRG and the national headquarters of Physicians for a National Health Program (which have shared office space for over two decades). I have worked closely with staff and board in many capacities, including serving as a spokesperson for the organization at public hearings, with the media, and at many of our conferences. It helps that I am a physician, because, for better or worse, the external world respects physicians. Fundraising, too, has been a part of my portfolio. I have always said, "You can't be serious about politics, if you're not serious about money."

Margie Schaps and I have shared an office for twenty years, plotting every day how to improve health and health systems, how to define work that HMPRG can do to make contributions, and how to strengthen our organization. I think Margaret Mead was right when she said: "Never doubt that a small group of thoughtful, committed (people) can change the world; indeed, it's the only thing that ever has."

John McKnight

John McKnight got to know Quentin in the 1950s and continues to have a close friendship with Quentin to this day. He retired from the Communication Studies Department at Northwestern University in 2005 and now serves as Emeritus Professor of Communication Studies.

I first met Quentin Young in 1956. We worked in the same building—he worked with the Chicago Board of Health and I with the Chicago Commission on Human Relations. We were both members of the Committee To End Discrimintion In Chicago Medical Institutions—a descriptive but unwieldy name for a small group of people working to end exclusion of African-American patients and doctors from service in Chicago hospitals.

Over the next 25 years, we continued to work together on issues related to inequity in medicine. By 1981, I had joined the Urban Affairs faculty at Northwestern University and Quentin was chair of the Department of Medicine at Cook County Hospital. In his reform efforts at the hospital, Quentin engaged in a long struggle with its administrative and political directors.

Friends of Quentin began to feel that he had done as much as he could in the hospital reform effort and that his prodigious talents could better be directed elsewhere. In discussion with these friends, I agreed to urge Quentin to resign from Cook County Hospital, and then we would create a new citizen oganization that could take on reform issues across the entire field of medicine. We developed a plan for the new organization. It would have at least 3 unique features.

First, the board would be comprised of diverse citizens who would not just set policy. They would also be the principal actors and advocates working on reform issues.

Second, the citizen board would set the agenda and not allow funders to influence the direction of the group. This meant we would need a lean staff and active board to minimize financial need.

Third, at that time, Quentin and I had worked in Cuernavaca, Mexico, with Ivan Illich, the radical critic and social historian. Illich emphasized that health was not the product of medicine. Rather, medicine was one of the numerous determinants of health and that it often misled people to believe there was something called a "health consumer." Illich argued that you could "consume" medicine but it was primarily the social, cultural and economic environment that "produced" health. For this reason, we decided the new organization should be primarily about health. The result was the marvelously unwieldy name—The Health and Medicine Policy Research Group or HMPRG for short. It is pronounced, by those in the know, "Humpurg."

Looking back, the three founding principles have served us well, and there is little doubt that HMRPG is now the most influential local citizen-run health advocacy group in the nation. Throughout all these years, the visionary leader and driving force has been Quentin Young.

Thirteen

May 25, 2011

Dear Rep. Paul Ryan,

Our organization, Physicians for a National Health Program, is strongly supportive of Medicare, recognizing it as one of the premier legislative achievements in the history of the United States. Therefore, I am writing to express our gratitude for your role in eliciting the overwhelming support that the people of our country extend to this important social justice program.

Since you succeeded in securing virtual unanimous support from the Republican majority in the House of Representatives for your voucher program, the rejection of your plan has been demonstrated nationwide. The spectacular defeat of Ms. Corwin in the 26th district of New York on May 24, 2011, is clearly the earliest expression of the vital importance our nation attaches to a single-payer comprehensive health plan for the elderly, Medicare.

I can think of no other political act that could match your voucher program "reform" in mobilizing public support for Medicare going forward. The collateral damage to the Republican aspirations for power is immeasurable.

Thank you very much,

Quentin Young, M.D., M.A.C.P
National Coordinator, Physicians for a National Health Program

cc: President Barack Obama, Speaker John Boehner

If you can't have a little fun while trying to change the world, why bother? Whether Paul Ryan—who as the Republican nominee for vice president a year later would be pushing the same plan to eviscerate Medicare—understood my sarcasm is debatable. Fortunately, he and his 2012 running mate, the shape-shifting Mitt Romney, never gained traction with the voucher argument, were rejected by the electorate, and Medicare survives... at least for now. But don't take that as a ringing endorsement of the Obama administration's health care policies.

The president and I go back a long way. He has been the patient of my partner Dr. David Scheiner. And I'm credited, or, equally often, discredited, with counseling him on the benefits of extending our successful Medicare program to cover everyone in the country. Just Google "Barack Obama" along with "Quentin Young" and see how many right-wing groups tried to tarnish him by associating him with me—the supposed communist and advocate for the "socialist" notion of single-payer, universal health care.

I'll get into my relationship with President Obama and my profound disappointment in Obamacare shortly. Before that, however, allow me to talk about the group that I referred to in my letter to Paul Ryan—the wonderful Physicians for a National Health Program (PNHP), a nationwide organization of doctors who have been advocating for a single-payer health care system for over a quarter of a century.

I admit to being prejudiced in terming it "wonderful." Its membership, which now exceeds 18,000, spans the country and includes some of the most dedicated, selfless and congenial doctors I've ever worked with. Our mission: "To educate physicians, other health workers, and the general public on the need for a comprehensive, high-quality, publicly funded health care program, equitably accessible to all residents of the United States."

Achieving such a program is a tall order, but the idea is simple, clear, and compelling in its logic.

I was present at the creation of PNHP in 1987 and have served as national coordinator since 1993. I've seen its membership and its state and city chapters multiply. Today, PNHP's national headquarters shares office space with HMPRG. If you are in Chicago and selling vowels, come visit us.

Some terminology. "Single-payer national health insurance" refers to a health system in which a single entity, usually a public agency, pays all medical bills. The delivery of care remains a mix of private and public providers. Think of it as an "improved Medicare for all," a system that operates much like Medicare operates for seniors today, a program which would automatically cover everyone in the country, from birth to death, according to the principle of "Everybody in, nobody out."

Or think Canada, for example. In my testimony before the House Committee on Ways and Means in 1991, I said, "PNHP looks to Canada, our close neighbor, for principles to rejuvenate our system. We wish to emulate, not mimic, the Canadian experience. There is every reason to excel here because we are wealthier."

I then enumerated some of its key principles, including universal, comprehensive, portable coverage for every inhabitant, the elimination of financial barriers to care, and public financing through equitable taxes amounting to less than what people pay now in premiums and out-of-pocket costs.

Shortly thereafter, appearing on ABC's "Nightline" with Ted Koppel, I put it his way: "Three reforms, real simple. Single-payer. What does that mean? National health insurance all going through a government payer. Sensible. Very simple. Negotiated fees with the doctors and other providers. We have to pitch in. And that's the law. In Canada, it's a felony if a doctor charges more than allowed on the provided services. And the doctors aren't doing badly, I assure you. Global budgets for the hospitals, and *voila*, a human system to replace this madness we've been talking about."

The "madness," of course, refers to our present arrangements in health care, which cost our patients and our society so much treasure and which inflicts such unnecessary suffering. Those arrangements stem from our dysfunctional, profit-seeking, private insurance firms and their allies: Big Pharma, the medical supply companies and for-profit hospitals.

Single-payer would change all this. By replacing the private insurers with a streamlined single-payer system, we can save over $400 billion squandered annually on administrative overhead, enough to cover all 50 million uninsured and eliminate co-pays and deductibles for everyone. Moreover, a single-payer system would, through its bargaining power, control costs and reduce our nation's deficit over the long term, a vital goal for our economy.

It's long overdue.

Although I was present for the birth of PNHP, I can't take credit for its conception. PNHP was the brainchild of a husband-and-wife team, Steffie Woolhandler and David Himmelstein, who proposed the organization to fellow clinicians in 1986. In an article on the early days of PNHP, the couple recalls being inspired by several factors, including a ballot initiative in Massachusetts that called on Congress to support single-payer reform, Reagan administration cuts to safety-net programs, and the success of Canada's single-payer program.

I would add that the laboratory conditions for the creation of PNHP were also right because the cost of health care was accelerating at an impossibly fast rate. One reason for the rise might be viewed as positive: the advent of interventions such as MRIs and bone marrow transplants that helped people combat disease. While life-saving, these were costly. But there was a bigger, more insidious reason for costs going through the roof: the ingress of for-profit insurance companies, which could control markets and in the process dictate costs for their own benefit.

I painfully remind you that physicians are very conservative. That's logical; they're small businessmen. But by the late 1980s, even doctors began to realize there was something worse than government, namely corporate control of the health system. Polls began to show these MDs were open to reform, including government sponsored insurance and the elimination of for-profit entities in the health system. The majority of these docs were not breast-beating supporters of single-payer like yours truly, but they were aware that the road they were traveling was hazardous for themselves and for their patients.

In their discussion of the beginnings of PNHP, Steffie and David note the contributions of Oliver Fein, Howard Waitzkin,

Gordy Schiff, Mardge Cohen, Henry Kahn, Jeff Scavron and Len Rodberg, and recall that by the end of 1987 about 200 dues-paying members had signed up. "From the outset," they write, "there was general agreement that the group should draw up a single-payer physicians' manifesto, with the hope that it could be published in a major journal, allowing us to increase our legitimacy and recruitment." In January 1989, the *New England Journal of Medicine* published just such a manifesto: "A National Health Program for the United States: A Physicians' Proposal."

Recruitment was also aided by an active cadre of PNHP leaders who gave speeches, wrote articles, and, when possible, gave testimony. That's still our m.o. after all these years.

In 1991, PNHP decided to move its headquarters from Boston to Chicago, which, as I've mentioned, is the locus of many national medical associations and, more importantly, Cook County Hospital. My dear friend from County, Dr. Ron Sable, took over as national coordinator.

Ron was already a legend in Chicago's LGBT community. In 1983 he and fellow County internist Dr. Renslow Sherer had founded the AIDS clinic at County that would eventually bear their names. He had also founded the AIDS Foundation of Chicago and IMPACT, a gay and lesbian political action committee. In 1987 he had become the first openly gay candidate to run for Chicago's City Council, narrowly losing.

Coping with the AIDS virus himself, Ron had cut back on his clinical work, but was able to provide strong leadership to the newly established Chicago headquarters that shared space with HMPRG. Sadly, he passed away at age 48 in 1993. That year, as his illness progressed, I assumed the role of national coordinator.

In my new, volunteer role I was aided by one of my partners in private practice, Claudia Fegan, along with Gordy Schiff at County and Ida Hellander, formerly of Public Citizen's Health Research Group.

Steffie and David write generously: "Quentin and Ida vastly increased PNHP's recruiting efforts and public visibility, turned our periodic meetings from small, informal affairs into well-organized, dynamic gatherings, and greatly facilitated membership communications. With help from Mike McCally, they secured grants from three foundations and tripled the budget."

They add, quite accurately, that Gordy and Claudia "both assumed an increasingly critical role in the organization, serving as PNHP presidents, traveling speakers, and unofficially helping to oversee the Chicago office."

When Bill Clinton was elected president in 1992, members of PNHP were generally optimistic, but clear-eyed. The former governor of Arkansas had campaigned on the promise to reform our health care system. However, his campaign plank on this issue reflected a distinctly pro-corporate bias, and at the time PNHP gave it a grade "D."

Sure enough, on taking office, the president created a task force chaired by first lady Hillary Clinton. The task? Come up with a plan for universal health care for all Americans.

Those of us in the single-payer camp had strong feelings about what that plan should look like. Vicente Navarro of Johns Hopkins, PNHP's first health policy director, sat on the task force and a number of PNHP representatives were afforded the opportunity to address it. They emphasized, of course, the merits of a single-payer national health insurance model.

Before the end of the year, the Clinton health plan was on the table. Like his original campaign plank, it was corporate-friendly and in many ways resembled a freshened-up version of Richard Nixon's health plan in the 1970s. It relied on similar principles: a mandate that employers provide health coverage to their employees or pay into a special fund ("play or pay"), and a privileged role for a handful of big insurers who would monopolize the market and push virtually all Americans into regulated private HMOs.

Once the Clinton plan was officially unveiled, PNHP examined and discussed its features once again. We found that our initial assessment of its flaws still held, and we took a clear stance to continue our single-payer advocacy.

The constraints Clinton's plan would have put on the insurance industry, as modest as they were, were still too much for that industry to contemplate. Working through various phony "coalitions," the insurers and corporate allies (including smaller health insurers who worried about being cut out of the picture) waged an all-out, well-financed campaign to defeat it.

Emblematic of this campaign were the famous "Harry and Louise" TV spots in which husband and wife talked at the kitchen table about the harm the bill was likely to do, the big "government bureaucracy" it would create, and so on. Those ads, combined with many other elements in this corporate-inspired campaign, ultimately led to the bill's defeat.

The fact that Hillary Clinton was in charge of the task force and that her way of doing business, for better or for worse, offended many people didn't help either. By the fall of 1994, the Clinton initiative was a goner.

PNHP immediately pressed the issue of single-payer reform once again. At the 1996 Democratic National Convention in Chicago, the Rev. Jesse Jackson and I joined doctors, nurses, labor leaders and citizens to demand the reinsertion of "universal health care" (admittedly not as definite as "single-payer") in the party's platform. The demand had been deleted by the platform committee in the weeks before. We held a four-day, round-the-clock vigil, getting both media and police attention.

State-based activism continued too. In 1997, my friend and patient Patrick Quinn, currently the governor of Illinois, called me and urged that we launch a campaign to amend Article 1 of the Illinois Constitution to declare decent health care as a fundamental right. Pat had been inspired by Joseph Cardinal Bernardin's 1995 pastoral letter in which he wrote, "Health care is an essential safeguard of human life and dignity, and there is an obligation for society to ensure that every person be able to realize this right."

We organized advisory referendums in dozens of political subdivisions of the state in 1998, 1999 and 2000, asking voters to call on the General Assembly to enact a plan to broaden health care coverage in the spirit of Cardinal Bernardin. All passed overwhelmingly, often by a margin of 10 to 1. But the Assembly refused to act.

So, on a blazingly hot August day in 2001, Pat and I laced up our hiking shoes and began walking from the Centennial Bridge spanning the Mississippi River in Rock Island, Ill. to Grant Park in Chicago—167 miles through towns, farmland, campuses, suburbs and inner-city neighborhoods. We averaged 12 miles a day.

Did our walk, which was often joined by supporters along the way, turn around the Assembly? Alas, no. But we heightened public awareness.

In 2001, I helped organize an extraordinary Washington hearing on universal, single-payer national health insurance featuring lawmakers such as Dennis Kucinich, John Conyers Jr., Barbara Lee and Donna Christiansen, who listened to testimony from Robert Reich, former secretary of labor, Dr. Marcia Angell, and about thirty other leading figures in medicine and health advocacy. The hearing was sponsored by the Congressional Progressive Caucus, Black Caucus, Hispanic Caucus and others, and helped set the stage for new legislative initiatives.

Recognizing that this was ultimately going to be a political decision by our national government or several states, we leapt at an invitation from Rep. Conyers, the longtime Democratic congressman from Detroit, to discuss meaningful legislation. Over the next several years, we worked with Rep. Conyers, Rep. Kucinich, congressional staffers, and others.

After several discussions with sympathetic lawmakers, including effective presentations from people in our ranks who were in the health finance field, we were charged with the task of writing a bill—a real, honest-to-God bill that would be entered into the Congress. And we did.

In 2003, Rep. Conyers and about two dozen co-sponsors introduced H.R. 676, then known as the U.S. National Health Insurance Act, now called Expanded and Improved Medicare for All Act. *Quelle surprise!* The bill was neither universally embraced nor enacted, but it immediately became an organizing tool for single-payer advocates nationwide.

God bless him, Congressman Conyers has continued to introduce the legislation every year since that time, and the number of co-sponsors has swelled to as many as 93 members of Congress. The bill has also been endorsed by more than 600 labor organizations and scores of civic and faith-based groups, not to mention the U.S. Conference of Mayors and over 60 municipal and county governments.

Unfortunately, H.R. 676 now sits in a House committee. The good news is that, thanks to the Congressional Black Caucus, the Progressive Caucus, and other so-called liberals, it retains a solid base of support.

So what, you ask, does H.R. 676 do? In short, it establishes a system of universal, single-payer health care paid for by taxes (as opposed to insurance premiums or, for those without insurance, out-of-pocket or "out-of-luck" payments). Our government would do what many governments in the civilized world do: pay for all legitimate, medically necessary care. *Adiós* private insurance companies. Hello public or not-for-profit institutions. Welcome to the ranks of the insured those thirty million of you who will remain uninsured under Obamacare.

The bill would provide all those residing in the U.S.—including noncitizens—with free health care, *a la* Medicare. Beyond primary and emergency care, this includes long-term health care; prescription drugs; mental health, dental, and vision services; and, importantly, prevention. Prevention not only benefits the individual patient, it benefits the system by keeping costs down. Individuals can choose their own doctors, clinics, and hospitals from those participating in the program—anticipated to be most health care providers.

How do we pay for this? In several ways: by redirecting the enormous sums we currently spend on wasteful, unnecessary, insurance-related paperwork and bureaucracy, estimated to be $400 billion annually, to clinical care; with monies already appropriated for Medicare, Medicaid, and other current appropriations for health care; and with modest taxes—on the very wealthiest, on payroll and self-employment earnings, and on stock transactions.

And how do we assure that the system works? By creating a board that monitors and makes recommendations concerning the accessibility, affordability, and quality of the care delivered. Besides, we have the successful track record of other nations' health systems—and our own Medicare program—to furnish sufficient evidence of the efficacy of this model.

The passage of the Affordable Care Act, or Obamacare, has

tended to push the discussion of single-payer reform to the sidelines. This unhappy development is why, quite frankly, I would have preferred to see Obamacare go down in defeat. It can be argued that the plan passed by Congress in March 2010 improved upon the status quo in several ways. But settling for what some characterized as "half a loaf" cost us the opportunity to get the full loaf. And it's only that full loaf—a single-payer system—that will solve our crisis in health care.

I wish the president had dug in and fought for more.

I first met the Barack Obama in the mid-1990s. If I'm not mistaken our earliest encounters were at the home of our mutual friend and East Hyde Park neighbor Linda Diamond Shapiro, who once served as the executive director of HMPRG. At the time, Obama was lecturing at the University of Chicago Law School and practicing law in the city. He was no longer a community organizer, but remained active in a number of community organizations. We did not become bosom buddies after a few of these social gatherings; I just viewed him as a nice, bright guy living in the neighborhood.

In 1996, the estimable Alice Palmer, who represented our Hyde Park/Kenwood community in the Illinois Senate, decided to run for Congress. She tapped Obama to run as her successor and introduced the fledgling politician to the community. One such introduction that I attended has become infamous: a breakfast at the home of one-time Weatherman Bill Ayers.

Watching Obama at this and similar gatherings, I was impressed. He was acquainted with the issues and, as we all know, a wonderful speaker. Here was an unusually skilled and informed young man. Our Hyde Park gang was happy that he was running and happy when he won.

I was happy with his views on health care, as well. He recognized that major reform was necessary and indicated support for a single-payer approach. No blushing friend, I took every opportunity to solidify this position. While not an official adviser, I tried to influence him as much I could. My colleagues and I sent him notes touting the advantages of single-payer and the form it might take and talked with him and his staff about it whenever I had the chance.

To be candid, I felt I did influence him. When he ran for the U.S. Senate in 2003, candidate Obama told the Illinois AFL-CIO: "I happen to be a proponent of a single-payer universal health care program. I see no reason why the United States of America, the wealthiest country in the history of the world, spending 14 percent of its gross national product on health care, cannot provide basic health insurance to everybody. And that's what Jim is talking about when he says everybody in, nobody out. A single-payer health care plan, a universal health care plan. That's what I'd like to see. But as all of you know, we may not get there immediately. Because first we've got to take back the White House, we've got to take back the Senate, and we've got to take back the House."

Still a state senator, in 2003, Obama sponsored the Health Care Justice Act. He made some comments that troubled me at the time. I'll let Dean Olsen a reporter for the Springfield-based *State Journal Register*, pick up the story:

"The legislation, just a few pages long, required the state to create a bipartisan committee to propose statewide reforms involving health care cost-containment and expanded access to comprehensive insurance coverage. But when House Bill 2268 passed the Democrat-controlled House in 2003 with a smattering of Republican votes, it contained a provision that the state, by 2007, would be required to implement a universal health care system.

The bill didn't give many specifics, but it was estimated such a system would cost the state $2.6 billion to $4 billion annually. The insurance industry feared the bill would institute a Canadian-style, single-payer system and result in many insurers going out of business.

Obama, who made statements in the early 2000s in support of a single-payer plan for the United States, agreed to remove the universal-care mandate after H.B. 2268 arrived in the Illinois Senate.

During a contentious floor debate when the bill passed the Senate on May 19, 2004, Obama said the House version was 'radically changed... in response to concerns that were raised by the insurance industry.'

According to the debate transcript, he also said the bill wasn't a 'Trojan horse' to introduce 'single-payer.' 'I want to say on record that I am not in favor of a single-payer plan,' he said. 'I don't think that we can set up that kind of plan, and if we were going to even attempt... some sort of national health care, that would have to, obviously, be done at the federal level.'

Dr. Quentin Young, a friend of Obama from Chicago, said he was impressed by Obama's commitment to health care reform as a young state lawmaker. But Young, national coordinator of Physicians for a National Health Program, was disappointed that Obama abandoned the single-payer plan. "We have single-payer for people over 65—it's called Medicare," Young said. "I was very disappointed by his move to the right to keep insurance companies in command. I'm not accusing him of lying or misconduct. I'm accusing him of a lack of courage."

In 2006, I was appointed by the president of the Illinois Senate to be a member of the Adequate Health Care Task Force, whose charge was to make recommendations for state reform. Six proposals came before our committee, including a single-payer proposal crafted by my PNHP colleagues. Although the single-payer plan earned the highest score from Navigant Consulting, which had been retained to evaluate the plans for such things as universality and cost, it was ultimately pushed aside in favor of a much weaker "Health Care Coverage Expansion Model." The influence of the private health insurers in this connection was palpable.

Under the "Expansion Model," all Illinois residents would be required to secure health insurance. Illinoisans who fell a certain percentage under the federal poverty level would be eligible for subsidies. Employers would be a major player—either by providing their workers with a voluntary health insurance plan or by paying the state an amount scaled to wages; again, "play or pay." Some new insurance regulations would also be imposed. In many ways, particularly the mandate and the subsidies for private insurance, it was similar to what we know as Obamacare.

Much of the plan became part of Gov. Rod Blagojevich's "Illinois Covered" legislation introduced later in 2007. That legislation died, thanks to opposition from the insurance industry, businesses that would have had to pay in, and Blagojevich haters on both sides of the aisle in Springfield—a considerable contingent.

**

Despite my disappointment in Barack Obama's lack of courage, I supported him when he ran for the U.S. Senate in 2004 and when he decided to run for president just a few years after winning that seat. His public pronouncements against the war in Iraq and for serious health care reform as well as my observation that he was a smart, savvy politician made him my guy. Again, during these campaigns, I was not an adviser, but, along with others in the health reform movement, I had a close relationship with many of his inner circle. We had every reason to believe that our viewpoint, if not our specific proposals, would get serious attention in the Obama camp.

The November 4, 2008, election results were cause for celebration. The precise conditions that Obama had spoken of in 2003 as necessary for passage of a single-payer plan—a Democrat in the White House and Democratic Party control of both the House and the Senate—now existed. Sadly, however, the new president further retreated from supporting a single-payer plan, saying it would be "too disruptive."

There were other signs of trouble, including his appointments of many Wall Street executives to his cabinet.

The president did push ahead on health reform. He issued a call for a large conference of lawmakers, health policy experts, and leaders of civic groups to hear their opinions. Among the initial group of invitees, there was not a single advocate for single-payer—even though many surveys have shown it enjoys solid majority support. Only after PNHP members and others threatened to picket outside the White House gates were PNHP President Dr. Oliver Fein and Rep. Conyers invited at the last minute. I was not personally invited, but in the receiving line, the president told Fein something like, "Give my regards to Quentin." It was a nice gesture, but it was no substitute for a serious discussion of an improved Medicare for all.

In fact, Max Baucus, a middle-of-the-road Democratic senator out of Montana who carried the ball on health care for the president in Congress, announced that everything was on the table—*except single-payer.* It took the civil disobedience of eight single-payer advocates, including Drs. Margaret Flowers and Carol Paris, in Baucus' hearing room to get a modicum of media attention to this scandalous omission.

What a gratuitous insult. You can keep something on the table and see if it goes anywhere. In my humble opinion, however, Baucus wanted to appease the insurance companies and HMOs that backed him—all those power groups that were spending millions to assure that there would be no progressive fundamental change in the American health system.

Call it pragmatism or lack of backbone, the president didn't push back against Baucus. Again, he had already repudiated his previous position. At a town hall meeting in Portsmouth, New Hampshire, in August 2009, he responded to a question as to whether he supported a universal health care plan:

"First of all, I want to make a distinction between a universal plan versus a single-payer plan, because those are two different things. A single-payer plan would be a plan like Medicare for all, or the kind of plan that they have in Canada, where basically government is the only person—is the only entity that pays for all health care. Everybody has a government-paid-for plan, even though in, depending on which country, the doctors are still private or the hospitals might still be private. In some countries, the doctors work for the government and the hospitals are owned by the government. But the point is, is that government pays for everything, like Medicare for all. That is a single-payer plan.

I have not said that I was a single-payer supporter because, frankly, we historically have had an employer-based system in this country with private insurers, and for us to transition to a system like that I believe would be too disruptive. So what would end up happening would be, a lot of people who currently have employer-based health care would suddenly find themselves dropped, and they would have to go into an entirely new system that had not been fully set up yet. And I would be concerned about the potential destructiveness of that kind of transition.

All right? So I'm not promoting a single-payer plan."

In March 2010, the decidedly non-single-payer Affordable Care Act passed Congress by a narrow margin. PNHP's policy experts did a line-by-line examination of the bill and, while acknowledging that it contains some modest benefits that make changes around the edges of our existing system, basically gave it two thumbs down. To this day, much to the chagrin of many of our friends who wanted reform, I remain adamant in my rejection of Obamacare.

Why? We want a system that excludes the private insurance companies. We demand such exclusion not because these companies are good or evil (although we think they're pretty evil). Rather, the reason to exclude them is that they don't address the needs of the American people. Giving a deductible of $2,000 before you get any benefit is Exhibit A. As a result, people don't get care early. They avoid seeking care because it costs them so much despite the insurance.

I want to stress that single-payer is not a "radical" idea. We have in this country since 1965 experience with that kind of insurance for the most costly sector of the population—people over 65 with all the attendant ills that come with age. No program that I know of is superior to Medicare in its popularity with the public.

I don't have any sympathy for the idea that the president had to compromise because his opposition was strong. Winning is not always winning the election. Winning is making a huge fight and then taking the fight to the people—reelecting people who are supporting your program and defeating those who aren't.

But you have to be prepared to struggle and the president seemed ready to give in from the beginning. So we have a dreadful situation. Had I been in Congress, I unequivocally would have voted against Obamacare. It's a bad bill. Whether it's worse than what we've got could be argued. We rather think because of its ability to enshrine and solidify the corporate domination of the health system, it's worse than what we have now. But whether it's somewhat better or a lot worse is immaterial. The health system isn't working in this country—fiscally, medically, socially, morally.

It's also important for me to note that the inclusion of a so-called public option would not have made any significant difference on the overall impact of this bill, contrary to the view of many progressives who believed it would. (My colleague Nicholas Skala argued this very point before the Congressional Progressive Caucus in 2009. Tragically, Nick, who was a very close friend, died in just a few months later at age 27.)

As you might guess, my stance on health care reform has not earned me any invitations to the White House. I don't take umbrage at that. The president has a lot more to worry about than an old friend who didn't support the signature legislation of his first term.

Paul Ryan's voucher system failed to gain any serious traction because the vast majority of Americans favor retention of Medicare. Approach its fiftieth birthday, it still works. So why shouldn't this happy experience with a single-payer, government-run health system be expanded to all Americans? On average our health costs in the U.S. are twice as expensive as the nineteen countries that have single-payer, and our statistics on wellness and longevity trail the single-payer nations.

We can't go on like this. This would be a challenge if the health system and economy were rich and not faltering, but they are faltering. That's one reason why we think that sooner rather than later politically it will be feasible to push for national health insurance and join the rest of the human race in maximizing the benefits of the health system.

This is not wishful thinking. Indeed some states are beginning to push in this very direction. Vermont has passed and the governor has signed a bill which declares single-payer to be its ultimate goal. During the battle over Obamacare and during the

2012 presidential election, we heard a number of politicians—the vast majority of the Republicans—argue that the fifty states should be "laboratories" for all kinds of different health care reform initiatives. While heartened by the approach in Vermont, PNHP remains steadfast in the belief that the most efficient and responsible approach is a nationwide system. That's more or less what Medicare does and it produces a very good product. Not the best—it could stand reform, too—but it is certainly better than private insurance.

Some in our country say, "Let the marketplace award care according to ability to pay." We rigorously reject that. Health care is a human right. There should not be market solutions in a life-and-death game.

Since WWII, we have learned a lot about disease and certainly have had dramatic improvements in what we can do. I'm talking about surgery on the heart, vaccination, nutrition issues. All these things have been largely defined in the last half-century. We've had something approaching a 12-year life expectancy rise just from scientific intervention.

We have all this knowledge, all these options, but we have a very backward financing and delivery system and the result is a great deal of human suffering. And that is why we remain opposed to the Affordable Care Act. We think we have a winning proposition despite the reality in Congress. Polls repeatedly vindicate our position. A solid majority of the public and 59 percent of doctors support the single-payer approach.

President Obama could have made it happen. He could have stuck to all the virtues of single-payer. And I won't deny he may have been defeated in the first round. There's no question that this fight has been dirty and it's going to get dirtier. For example, calling single-payer national health insurance "socialized medicine," as many lawmakers and pundits have, isn't even a cheap political term. It's a lie.

Single-payer national health insurance isn't socialized medicine. It's organizing your system the way much of the rest of the world has. It's recognizing that health care is a human right and acting accordingly.

Claudia Fegan
*Claudia Fegan trained at Michael Reese where she first en-
countered Quentin Young in her professional career in 1982. She
practiced with Quentin from 1988 until 2000 when she left private
practice to work for the Cook County Health and Hospital System
where she currently serves as the Executive Medical Director for the
System.*

I joined Quentin in practice on October 1, 1988, and attended my
first PNHP meeting the following spring. Each meeting was such an
energizing event; physicians brought together from around the country
discovered they were not alone in realizing there is something terribly
wrong with health care in the United States. At first it was a few dozen,
but the numbers have steadily grown to today, where hundreds attend.
We leave each meeting enthusiastic to carry forward the struggle for
single-payer.

When PNHP members gather, they talk about events they have
held locally in the fight to win equal access to health care. They talk
about different tactics they have used, efforts to raise funds, ways to
get media coverage and successes in reaching large numbers of people. People always look forward to these meetings as opportunities to
connect with fellow comrades in the struggle for health care justice, a
chance to see the latest version of the updated slideshow by David and
Steffie and of course, a chance to hear from Quentin.

David Himmelstein and Steffie Woolhandler developed a compelling set of slides (it used to be a set of Kodachrome slides, now it is a
PowerPoint presentation) filled with data about the injustice of health
care in this country. It is used by PNHP members to educate the public
about the need for single-payer health care.

At some point during the meeting people look to Quentin to tell us
how we are going to get this done. Members have their own ideas on
strategy and have been actively engaged in this struggle throughout the
year, but Quentin is the sage elder statesman. Maybe he is our Yoda,
he has weathered movements for civil rights and for human rights and
we believe he will help get us there.

Quentin was in his mid-60's when PNHP started over 25 years
ago; now many of those once youthful founders are crossing that
threshold. Always a visionary, Quentin was never wedded to the status
quo, even though he was part of the medical establishment. He was
never afraid of change and attracted young people who wanted to make
a difference. Quentin never told us what to do, but was supportive and
encouraging.

When I was a small child, I knew of Quentin because he was regarded with reverence by my parents because of his positions on civil rights and worker causes. I had encountered Quentin during my residency training at Michael Reese. As a result of all of his advocacy work, he often showed up at the hospital in the evenings to see his patients. He was always quite conversational at those times, and never missed the opportunity to extrapolate the plight of a patient who presented with a late diagnosis to the suffering of the masses and how this country's failure to provide access to decent health care is killing people. It was seldom about the individual, it was the application of the plight of the individual to the plight of society and its workers. With his help, I learned the aspect of Medicine that medical education fails to include, but is so crucial if you are going to practice medicine and make a difference.

Fourteen

While much of my time over the past thirty-plus years has been devoted to advancing the worthy initiatives of HMPRG and PNHP, there have been many other people, places, and platforms that have captured my heart or mind, or both. Harold Washington. Michael Reese. Cook County Hospital. APHA. WBEZ. Cuba and Sudan. And my darling Ruth.

Let's start with Harold, the first African American to be elected mayor of Chicago, one of the most racially divided cities in the world. Around the time Harold beat then Mayor Jane Byrne and future mayor Richard M. Daley in the Democratic primary in 1983, I called him "the most rounded, elegant politician I've ever known." That holds true today some 25 years after his untimely death in November 1987.

Beginning in 1965, Harold had been Hyde Park's man in Springfield, serving first as a state representative and then as a state senator. In 1980, he had become our U.S. congressman. Our paths had crossed both socially and professionally. While at County I had lobbied for his support of the hospital and a variety of community health initiatives. He was a progressive, to be sure. Still, as a precinct captain's son and as an aide to the Daley-connected ward boss Ralph Metcalfe, he knew the Machine well.

Before officially entering the race for mayor, Harold appeared before a number of community groups to gauge potential support. I remember chairing a large meeting and pushing him to commit. "Mr. Washington, you informed your base that you wouldn't run unless they registered 100,000 people, and the latest number shows they've registered 150,000. Are you going to try to bow out because they registered *more* than you wanted?"

Shortly after that, when he had committed to run, Harold received the enthusiastic endorsement of a well-informed citizen who had previously exhibited, shall we say, a cynical attitude towards politicians. My second wife Ruth (much more about her later) had to entertain Harold in our home while I took a phone call. One-on-one the politician charmed her as he charmed almost everyone he met. "I love him," Ruth whispered to me upon my return. He had won her over by demonstrating a scientist's knowledge of a subject dear to her heart, nuclear energy. He was like that—able to expound wisely on almost any topic.

On the eve of the primary, which everyone knew would determine who would become mayor in our overwhelmingly Democratic city, I wrote a lengthy op-ed piece in the Chicago *Tribune* urging voters to choose Harold. After noting that Mayor Byrne had "tapped into the public passion for something better and different" than what the Daleys represented, I lamented the fact that she "went on to kill that dream." It was still politics as usual at City Hall and "there is no aspect of government, from public health services to public safety that is not in disarray."

Why Washington? "His intelligence, wit, and wisdom... are harmonious companions to his uncommon passion and remarkable leadership. Clearly the man is a political healer for these morbid times... He has begun the emancipation of the black community from the thralldom of machine patronage domination, an immeasurable gain for everyone and a model for other sectors... Washington's long public record on issues vital to labor, to the peace movement, to civil libertarians, to the elderly, to women, is exemplary. In all of these efforts he has been color blind."

Of course, the Chicago electorate has never been color blind. Harold did garner a significant number of votes from progressive whites, but he benefitted greatly because he was the lone black candidate running against two white contestants. He won the primary with 37 percent of the vote. Byrne received 33 percent, while Daley took 30 percent. In the general election he prevailed over another Hyde Parker, former state representative Bernard Epton, by a slim 51.7 percent to 48 percent margin.

In seeking to become the first Republican mayor since 1931,

Epton, a one-time civil rights advocate, seemed willing to compromise his principles. His slogan, (with which he was said to be uncomfortable, but nevertheless approved) was, "Epton—before it's too late."

Not very subtle, but effective. Epton received 81 percent of the white vote (but only 3 percent of the black vote). Several Democratic ward organizations and prominent Machine figures also backed him. Their opposition would continue after the election, making it difficult for Harold to govern at all, much less institute reforms that needed City Council approval.

After the election, Harold created a transition team to analyze the major issues confronting the city and to make recommendations on how to proceed. Along with Dr. Robert Stepto, of the University of Chicago Pritzker School of Medicine, I chaired the Health and Human Services Policy Task Force. "Study calls city health services 'in disarray,'" read a front page *Tribune* headline in July 1983 after we released our report.

What did we recommend? Reorganize the Department of Health, create agencies on women's affairs and human rights, and create a new body to coordinate and monitor the city's efforts, the Health and Human Services Council. The *Tribune*'s Tim Franklin reported: "In calling for restructuring of the health department, Young lashed out at its management under past administrations: 'It abandoned the commitment that was a long tradition of the city to public health. It became... perhaps the pre-eminent example of patronage politics. Time and again we saw people placed in posts at the behest of elements outside the department to meet political needs.'"

Be careful what you wish for. Our task force suggested replacing some of those people at their posts. And soon Harold appointed me president of the Chicago Board of Health. (The City Council held up the appointment along with more than a dozen other ones. During my tenure, I was "acting president.") This appointment offered no salary, but the potential for effecting change was significant. By statute the board serves as chief health policy adviser to the mayor. The mayor then turns to the Department of Health to carry out what he or she decides upon. The Department is run by a full-time, salaried commissioner.

As the previous chapters indicate, I had observed and fought the Machine on numerous occasions. I knew City Hall well from the outside. But, I confess that battle-tested as I was, I did not appreciate the breadth and depth of the powers that be and had long been. During the three, sometimes four, days a week I spent at the job—I was also maintaining my private practice and going to the Health and Medicine office when I was able (certainly less than I had in the past)—I was inundated by visitors who complained about the way business had been conducted under past administrations and the newly installed Washington administration. The reorganization of the Health Department called for by our task force was sorely needed.

At one of my regular meetings with the mayor, I told him what I was hearing: "Everybody is coming in and telling me about the corruption and the malfeasance. Harold, you know I'm a cynic, but I can't believe it."

"Quentin," he said, "it's worse than you know."

After about a year I did know. I was continually stymied by the commissioner of health, who refused to cooperate or share information. I can only speculate that he was in over his head or knew exactly what he was doing, but felt cooperating would result in his own loss of power.

I shared the problem with Harold and told him I wanted to resign in a way that would not bring any embarrassment to his administration. At first he refused to accept the resignation, but soon he relented. He had bigger issues to worry about. There were more than a few less-than-competent administrators at City Hall. Harold himself was a remarkably principled, highly intelligent man and I enjoyed every moment I worked with him. But that doesn't mean everybody in his entourage was such. And he knew it.

Three years after I left, little had changed according to the president of the Board of Health, my old friend from County, Dr. Jorge Prieto. The department has " been in bad shape for decades, but it's far worse than it was in 1983," he told the *Tribune*. "We have to start taking care of the poor and we're not doing that." He explained that he didn't blame Harold, but, rather the mayor's "palace guard" which prevented him from having input on the mayor's policies.

The *Trib*'s John Kass explained that complaints of this nature "made privately by Prieto to his colleagues were of the same kind made more than three years ago by Young." Kass also noted that HMPRG, as well as Prieto, had voiced unhappiness with the state of affairs at the city's community clinics; it took as long as four months before pregnant women could be seen at these facilities.

My dissatisfaction with the city's delivery of health services while I was at the Board of Health and at HMPRG raises the question: Was I happier and more effective inside or outside of city government? By and large, I have been an outsider, and the relationship you have when you're not part of the establishment allows for a level of freedom of motion and expression that you don't have when you're part of the administration and confined by other considerations.

In this particular instance, because Harold had so many detractors and opponents, health was a lower priority for him so I couldn't get the attention paid to health in order to make the changes we needed. So I felt I could be more effective working through Health & Medicine to effect change than being part of the administration. This did not diminish or limit the support for Harold's agenda which I totally embraced.

Harold won a second term by a convincing margin in April 1987. Seven months later, on the day before Thanksgiving, he died of a heart attack at his desk. It was a sad day for Chicago. He was a remarkable politician, and he would have had much smoother sailing in the coming years with more citizens supporting him and fewer aldermen obstructing him.

One week after Harold's death, the *Tribune* published my op-ed piece titled, "A Health Care System to Honor Harold Washington." Here I opined that a comprehensive health care system could be "fashioned into a glorious homage to the man and his vision." Such a system would include a new, leaner Cook County Hospital with fewer beds and more community clinics—a plan our 1983 transition committee had suggested, that Harold had endorsed, and which the Cook County Board of Commissioners were currently proposing. "As (Washington) emerged from the council-fettered first term, he saw the possibilities, at long last, of bringing the counterproductive, wasteful and dysfunctioning turfs of city, county, university, and state health enterprises into harmony."

Fifteen years after Harold's death, a new, lean County Hospital opened its doors across the street from the old, sprawling edifice. This incarnation was not named after our deceased mayor, but, rather, a long-time County commissioner and board president. John J. Stroger Jr. Hospital has 434 beds and is part of a network that includes many of the elements proposed for years by HMPRG as well as the recommendations of that 1983 Health Task Force. This network included a revamped Provident Hospital, Oak Forest Hospital, the County Jail health service, and community clinics and a primary academic affiliation with nearby Rush Medical College, as well as minor affiliations with Chicago Medical School, Chicago College of Osteopathic Medicine, and the University of Illinois College of Medicine.

A timeline: Provident, which long served Chicago's African American community, had closed in 1987. Three years later the county had purchased the property from the federal government and committed millions to renovation and upgrading. The hospital had reopened in 1993.

A year later, County, which had lost its accreditation between 1991 and 1992, had affiliated with Rush. Around the same time in 1994, the Illinois Health Facilities Planning Board approved construction of a new hospital. In 1998, the County Board had approved the contract to build a new hospital and held a ground-breaking ceremony which I attended.

In his book, *County*, David Ansell rightly describes another Ruth, Ruth Rothstein, as the coalition-builder who made the new hospital possible. Ruth had been a labor organizer before taking over the reins at Mt. Sinai Hospital. After replacing the Machine's George Dunne as County Board president in 1990, Richard Phelan had wisely tapped her to run the hospital. After restoring County's accreditation, she turned her attention to getting approval and funding of a new facility. Ansell writes:

"She positioned herself at the center of the campaign. She assembled a civic coalition of some of the most prominent A-list individuals... After months of tours of the old hospital and meetings with editorial boards, the corner was turned... Years of demonstrations and strikes, against all odds, with a wall of opposition from the *Tribune*, the private hospitals, and most of Chicago's political leadership were over... Ruth Rothstein had pushed, nodded, and prodded until she got what we all wanted and what the patients needed—a new County Hospital."

I concur. I had known Ruth for years and I was part of this civic coalition working to establish the case for the new hospital—watching Ruth navigate this difficult task was most impressive. At one point she had trained as a lab technician in my offices. Her work at Sinai had been extraordinary and she deserves great credit for navigating the tricky terrain necessary to get a new County Hospital. She was a pragmatist who threaded the needle by accommodating the political powers that be—a necessity—without making the hospital a satellite of the Democratic Party. (Kudos, too, to her deputy, Pat Terrell, the first executive director of HMPRG.)

The dedication in 2002 was momentous. This was a remarkable achievement at a time of reducing public hospitals in this country. A brand new, modern facility dedicated to caring for the poor was finally available. At the dedication John Stroger acknowledged that Health & Medicine had played a key role in achieving this reality. Despite the fact that John was a very important part of the Democratic Party control of public health, we nonetheless had a respectful and cooperative relationship.

While my beloved Cook County Hospital has enjoyed a somewhat happy evolution, the same cannot be said of another one of my old stomping grounds, Michael Reese Hospital. Reese, founded in 1881, filed for Chapter 11 bankruptcy in 2008 and is no more. At its height it boasted 2,400 beds; when it closed it had only 150.

Reese's demise was in part attributable to changing demographics and deteriorating infrastructure. But there's another villain in this story: the for-profit health care model.

Another timeline: despite being financially viable, Reese is sold to Humana in 1991. Within three years it is part of the Columbia/HCA health network. Remember those guys? HCA, the largest private health care provider in the world, was founded by the Frist family of Tennessee in 1968. Dr. Bill Frist, son of the founder, was at one time U.S. Senate majority leader. The company went public in 1969, and twenty years later Frist's father took it private in a $5.3 billion buyout.

In the late 1990s things got interesting. 1997: the FBI serves search warrants on the company and doctors. CEO Rick Scott resigns in the face of scandal (He's now the Republican governor of Florida!). In 2000 and 2002, the company reaches settlements on fourteen felony counts, paying over $800 million for overcharging the government, bilking Medicare, kickback arrangements, and other fraudulent activities. It paid the same or more in civil claims, too.

There's much more, but let me focus on one event. In 2005 Senator Frist and other HCA executives sold shares in advance of a disastrous earnings report. Insider trading? Shareholders thought so, sued, and recovered $20 million. I should note that during its difficulties, HCA sold Reese to another company, Envision Healthcare.

When Humana bought Reese, I told the New York *Times* that, "Humana would reduce teaching programs and indigent care and was likely to close the hospital if operating losses persisted."

The big money guys disagreed. "I'd be surprised if they closed the hospital," Kenneth S. Abramowitz, an analyst with Sanford C. Bernstein & Company, told the newspaper. Maybe I should have worked on Wall Street.

Here's what I saw twenty years ago and continue to see: a commodity-driven arrangement that encourages marketplace instead of humanitarian solutions. Today we have a system of competitive agencies and hospitals. Years ago there were few for-profit hospitals. In Chicago, private groups of citizens would see the need for a hospital in their respective communities and build it:

Swedish Covenant, Illinois Masonic, Mount Sinai, Mercy.

The hospitals were a civic creation and had a social compact with the government, from which they'd get tax breaks, subsidies and urban renewal. In addition, they received support from local citizens grateful for round-the-clock emergency services and care. The system was responsive and community-based.

Enter the current for-profit status of hospitals, and you have a complete distortion and undermining of this once wholesome civic arrangement. Most of HCA's hospitals in this country were bought, not built, at marked-down prices as they struggled to make ends meet.

HCA and others bought public and private hospitals, forgoing the tax-free status for profits. This has not been a happy moment for American patients. Each one of these hospitals must make a profit, and not just any profit, a certain level of profit determined by the corporation. These companies and their stockholders operate on the premise that if there isn't a profit of 10, 12, 15 percent, the hospital should be closed down and money put where they can get a good return.

The for-profits have done a number of things to distort the market of health care. First and foremost, they cherry-pick patients who are well. Second, they often cheat, as in the case of HCA outlined above. Sadly, nobody ever goes to jail. They just pay these fines, smile, go into their treasury, and get fined again.

No one should be smiling. These fines are for egregious behavior, for criminally exceeding the allowed Medicare payment. When you're getting these fines, you've violated en masse. The government doesn't just come in and fine you $1 million for a $10 overcharge. The government audits and finds that you have been systematically overcharging, and in that way distorting the system.

While I'm on my soapbox, I should note that the profit motive of the drug companies isn't doing us any favors either. The pharmaceuticals justify charging huge amounts of money for prescription medications because they put so much money into research and development and they have a lot of losers along the way. They argue that if they don't charge that much for some of these drugs, they won't engage in research and development. I think that is a largely specious argument.

In truth, the drug companies throw everything, including the kitchen sink, into the cost of developing drugs, when much of what they claim as the cost of development is the cost of marketing and publicizing. I think the Big Pharma has been greedy in many ways, some of them quite startling. For example, some drugs have bad outcomes, but the companies are not required to make that public. More than once they have marketed these drugs, or at least kept from the distributors the facts about them.

These companies march to a different drummer—namely profit-seeking—and I'm very concerned that they profit mightily, not from their own "costly" research, but from research that's conducted by institutions. They profit by patenting the drug under their rubric and then they fight to extend the period of time for which their patent exists, as opposed to letting a drug go generic and cost much less.

In case you can't tell, let me say it: I am not optimistic about the development of medication by the profit-seeking sector, by the corporate entities. They just have a different motivation. And when they do what they're supposed to do, the public is not necessarily well served. They get drugs that are harmful, they get drugs that are not effective, they get drugs that are useful but cost a lot because they're patented.

So what, in the idealistic world of Quentin Young, is the motivator to stimulate continued research for drugs and other technologies to treat disease and illness if it's not the profit motive? In my utopia, the research and marketing and distribution of the drugs that are worthwhile is done by the government The drugs are developed by scientists who are not motivated by corporate greed, but by the application of their work. Look at the winners of the Nobel Prize in Medicine; these people are not profit-seekers. It's much more common for the scientific victories to take place in the not-for-profit sector—medical schools and research institutions—as opposed to the for-profit results in the industry. (And by the way, I do think people who make brilliant discoveries should get rewarded, whether it's a fraction of the patent return or something else, but I don't think that giving the incentive to for-profit drug companies is the way to go. It's one of the important causes of our runaway costs in health care.)

This book would be incomplete if I didn't mention two more important institutions that literally encompass the alphabet—from APHA to WBEZ. APHA is the American Public Health Association, a Washington, D.C.-based organization with a membership of over 25,000 health care workers. Founded in 1872, its mission is to "protect all Americans and their communities from preventable, serious health threats and strive to assure that community-based health promotion and disease prevention activities and preventive health services are universally accessible in the United States."

The public health sector is always subordinate to the private and corporate sectors in this country (the AMA, the insurers, Big Pharma, etc.). APHA offered a way for the public sector to speak with a united voice on behalf of the public's health. I was privileged to be the Association's president in 1988 and am still a proud, card-carrying member and participant in conferences and the like.

A look at APHA's policy statements adopted at its January 2013 meeting indicates the breadth of issues and the sensibilities. We've taken progressive stands on increasing physical activity among Americans; taxing sugar-sweetened beverages; curtailing military recruiting in public schools; improving occupational and environmental conditions in the global electronics industry; calling for increased public health capacity to monitor, regulate and respond to fracking in local communities; improving management of modern environmental insults to address emerging pollutants, failing infrastructure, climate change and industrial operations; calling for incorporating occupational information in electronic health records because the work environment has a well-recognized influence on health through exposures to physical, chemical and other hazards as well as stress and other working conditions that can be detrimental to health; protesting the disruption of public health and safety in immigrant communities; proposing changes to the regulations that govern ethics, safety and oversight of human research; calling for health impact assessments to be institutionalized at the federal, state and local levels; calling for regulations with respect to the use of mercury by dentists; and calling for increased overdose education. And that's just 2013!

APHA also organizes trips abroad. Cuba has been on the itinerary for many years. The association rightfully has a friendly attitude towards our island neighbor's health endeavors. Here is an impoverished country with monumental, exemplary health achievements reflected by life expectancy, birth, and infant mortality statistics.

I went to Cuba in the early 1970s as part of an APHA delegation. We stayed close to the ground, meeting with doctors and organizations. Doctors were to be found in virtually every Havana neighborhood and into all of rural Cuba. Access to health care was easy and prompt. There was a heavy emphasis on preventive medicine—immunization and such. Cuba had quite a good deal of accomplishment in synthesizing medication and vaccinations.

We came to observe, not practice. We wanted to see and understand the organization of a heralded and recognized system. The fact that we had come from the richest country in the world to one of the poorest to see how *everyone* received really good care and benefitted from a fine prevention program was not lost on us or our hosts. (Not too long ago, I returned to Cuba with a group from PNHP. I found that the health system has held up and remains a point of pride for the government. Cuba has health missions across the world.)

On behalf of APHA, Physicians for Human Rights, the American Association for the Advancement of Science (AAAS), the American College of Physicians, and the Committee on Health and Human Rights of the Institute of Medicine, I also traveled to Sudan in May of 1990. Led by Eric Stover of AAAS, I was tasked to lobby for the release of a doctor sentenced to death by the Sudanese government. This doctor and other doctors and scientists were in jeopardy following a 1989 coup by Lieutenant General Omar Hassan Ahmad al-Bashir. The new pro-Islamist military government had banned independent newspapers, closed down political parties, and abolished unions and professional associations of lawyers, doctors, and other professionals.

Many opponents of this regime, including doctors, had been imprisoned. One doctor had been reported to have been tortured to death in April. Our mission was to win clemency for Dr. Mammoun Mohammed Hussein, a Khartoum gynecologist sentenced to hanging for organizing a strike. A fellow strike-organizing doctor had been given a fifteen-year sentence.

Eric and I first flew to Great Britain, where Amnesty International briefed us. Then it was on to Khartoum. Fortunately, by the time we arrived in Sudan, each doctor had been granted a presidential pardon and released. Apparently, because we were approaching Ramadan, the traditional time for clemency, al-Bashir was in a generous mood. Add to that domestic and international pressure and you have a happy ending. The other doctor would eventually come to America.

We had the opportunity to meet the doctors, who thanked us for our efforts.

Then we went to the American Embassy, where the ambassador was under the impression that the doctors were still in prison and that there was no way to save them. When we informed him that the doctors were already free, the ambassador was miffed that his own people didn't have that intelligence.

A word about the need for organizations like Physicians for Human Rights, Doctors Without Borders, and the like. These medical groups have encouraged American doctors and the American public to be aware of health problems in underdeveloped countries and they play an important role in meeting health care needs and indirectly impact international policy-making.

WBEZ, Chicagoland's public radio station, also fulfills an important role in the community and nationally, for that matter, as the home of both Ira Glass's *This American Life*, and the popular current events quiz show, *"Wait Wait Don't Tell Me."* For years, I had a regular show and was these station's medical contributor, speaking to the issues of the day, interviewing policymakers, and taking listeners' phone calls. For a time, my show was from 6 p.m. to 7 p.m.—they call this drive time—once a week; later my show was on weekday mornings. The board members of Health and

Medicine assisted in the production of these shows which lasted many years.

The offer to host came out of the blue. The station wanted to do regular one-hour shows on different subjects, including health. I had a pretty high profile at the time, so I was tapped. Noting that many in the listening area regarded me as an agitator, I asked if there would be any topics or opinions off limits. Told I would have free rein, I accepted. After more than a half century out of radio, I was back!

The show was not hard to do. I had plenty to talk about, so the need to prepare was minimal. We'd respond to medical issues in the news, say the need for immunization, or something happening, say a flu epidemic. Most of the guests were from Chicago, but we sometimes spoke with experts from other cities.

There are a lot of subjects that are controversial in contemporary medicine, as they should be because the final word isn't in. We'd have a panel of people on, say, whether or not to immunize everybody or what age should be excluded. How hard do you encourage people to get immunization? A full array of questions around a particular controversial topic.

I plead guilty to trying to get social issues in the mix. We had a segregated health system in Chicago. Most hospitals were more or less lily white, while a few took only people of color. We often spoke about that. We took calls after the first half hour and had plenty of people calling in and expressing themselves.

Occasionally there were some light moments. Once, we were talking with a pediatrician who had written an article opposing circumcision. He wasn't questioning circumcision as a religious act, but rather the conventional wisdom that the operation is a good preventive measure against disease.

Listeners called in their opinions. One lady hesitated for what seemed an eternity and then stated that circumcision made sex better.

I didn't hesitate. "Thank you ma'am. Next question?"

After about five years, programming changed and I became a contributor on other shows. Funny thing: Although I was on air much less frequently, people would assure me that they listened to me every day.

And now my Ruth. She was a lifelong Hyde Parker, but our paths never crossed until we met in 1978. We married in 1980. And we were together for the next 27 years until her untimely death in 2007. Those dates do not tell our love story.

Ruth was referred to me as a patient in 1978 for some minor ailment that I don't remember. She was a mature, University of Chicago-type, fifteen or so years my junior, married with two children. As with most patients, I tried to impress her with my clinical skills and to strike up an interesting conversation—in this case by showing her a book from our mutual alma mater, the U. of C. She, however, was not interested in chitchat. I treated her and soon learned she had overcome the ailment. End of Act One.

Six or seven months later, our practice receptionist informed that a Mrs. Weaver was on the line. I didn't remember a Mrs. Weaver, but picked up the phone.

"Dr. Young, are you married?" the woman on the other end asked.

"No."

"Do you have a significant other?"

I thought a little bit on that one. "No, not really. Who is this?"

"Ruth Weaver. I was your patient some months ago. My husband and I are separating and we're going to get divorced and we have these tickets to the symphony series and I wondered if you would be free to go."

I wasn't prepared for that. I really had no relations with patients—not because I'm such a moralist, but because it just never happened. It's a big taboo. I had no experience with this. And I didn't remember a Mrs. Ruth Weaver.

"When is the concert?" I shouldn't have even asked that. I should have in a nice way said I wasn't free.

"In October."

This was, perhaps May. The lady planned ahead! Hoping she'd get the point that I wasn't that interested, I said, "Why don't you call me closer to the date."

We left it at that. Months passed and there was another call.

"Ms. Wheeler is on the line," is how I heard it.

"Yes, Ms. Wheeler," I said.

"It's Weaver!" she said angrily. "I want to inform you of the date of the concert. It's this Saturday."

So I'm in trouble. I can't expect her to get a substitute in a week. Still... "What's the program?" I asked.

"It's Larry Adler. You don't know who he is. He's a classical harmonica player."

"Yeah, I know who he is." Adler had been an outspoken critic of the communist hunters at HUAC after World War II. Black-listed, he had moved to England in order to make a living. Now, he was a world-renowned artist. I agreed to go with Ms. Weaver.

So that was the start of Ruth. She had worked her entire adult life, and at this point was managing editor of the *Bulletin of the Atomic Scientists*, a prominent anti-nuclear bomb publication. The evening at the concert went well and soon we were seeing each other regularly and exclusively.

Less than a year after we began dating, I went to a conference in Rome. I called Ruth every day. During one of our chats, she said, "I want you to move in with me."

"What?" I informed her that only married people lived together.

"Well my kids are both away at school, so there'd be no problem with living together. But if you want I'll move in with you."

We went back and forth on this. I told her I had made the vow never to marry again. She said we'd have to break up. Wow! Nobody had ever said that to me. So I wisely said we could talk about this when we met up in England in a few days.

When we got off the phone, I started thinking I might lose her. In London, I popped the question, expecting nothing but joy on her part. To my surprise she said, "I don't want to get married."

What! "Wait a minute. I just offered my hand."

Eventually I prevailed and we married on New Year's Day 1980. Over the next 27 years, she co-opted me into community gardening, she worked with a local community group called Vigil Against Violence, we traveled to Stratford for Shakespeare, and she left the *Bulletin* and took over a wonderful literary magazine, *Primavera*.

In mid-2006, Ruth became ill. She was diagnosed with cancer of the ureter (that connects the kidney and bladder). She had all the diagnostic and therapeutic interventions and the care she got was okay, but it was a lost cause when it was finally diagnosed. She was a longtime smoker, and I don't know whether that was the underlying cause of her illness.

The cancer was tragic in its aggressiveness, quickly disabling her. There was one nice part of that if you can use the word nice. Toward the end of her life, we went to Stratford and she had a real remission. We were very aggressive there. We had always done two plays a day, and she stood the course. There are a few really nice places to eat and we went there and she ate. But when that was over, it was her last hurrah. She perished in January 2007. That was the end. There was no protracted dying.

There's a world of difference between being a patient or the spouse of a loved one and being a physician who has a lot of judgments to make. As a "civilian," I've worked very hard at being the patient or the patient's husband—taken off my lab coat. It doesn't always work. Today when I see my doctor, who's a very good doctor, he has a tendency to make me his consultant. And I don't want that. With Ruth, I obviously saw the decisions that various doctors were making. I don't mean to imply that I'm without any emotional investment. Quite the contrary. But I tried to be the patient's spouse rather than the doctor's consultant.

In Ruth's case I don't think it was a very complicated role to play. Her illness, once discovered and identified where it had spread, allowed little leeway. There were certain necessary interventions and they were taken. There's no denying that if your loved one has a lethal cancer, it affects you. You can't escape it and you don't want to escape it. It's quite something to go through. Certainly it concentrated my attention. To be candid, I still have subordination to that reality: the fact that at the end of the day we really couldn't do anything.

It's one thing with respect to providing the proper medical

treatment and knowing you can or can't do something, but there's a whole other way about how the news is broken to people. I have addressed that question as a doctor rather than as a patient's husband, and I have an explicit view of that. The important professional responsibility is to answer the patient's question and no more. It is understandable and positive that doctors are concerned about their patients. Sometimes, however, we are emotionally involved more than we really should be. The point is that you should listen to the patient's question or comment and respond to that.

Let's say we know that this patient has a cancer that's spread throughout the body. It's all identified and a matter of record. So the patient asks you, "Do I have cancer?" The answer is yes. But not yes and it's going to kill you in three weeks. That wasn't what the patient asked about. I've worked hard to teach younger doctors the idea that you should respond, but respond to the specific inquiry. Patients will stop asking questions when they can't take any more. Later they may ask some more.

I think I can claim that we sort of did that with Ruth. We knew all too well what everything was and were prepared to not conceal it or lie or not tell her the truth, but to give her what she could handle at the time. I wasn't her doctor mind you, but I was her husband who was a doctor. And I believe it worked pretty well. There's no way to make nice a fatal cancer. It's totally bad and catastrophic, but how you reveal that to the patient makes a difference.

When Ruth died, the *Tribune* interviewed my old friend Studs Terkel for the obituary: "With Ruth, (Quentin) met the perfect mate, they were a marvelous combination. She knew everything he was doing and, like a doctor, she felt, she had a feeling tone, a feeling for the other person. It was a great love story."

Amen.

Epilogue

My dear Ruth once told me that when she was twelve years old, she refused to take Communion, courageously telling her parents that she didn't believe in God.

In keeping with Jewish law, I was bar mitzvahed at age thirteen, but it wasn't long thereafter that I arrived at the same conclusion. I don't recall making a big deal about it, as Ruth did, but I do remember my outlook underwent a profound and lasting change.

That doesn't mean that I suddenly lost a sense of purpose or a moral center in my life. Quite the contrary. From my adolescent years to the present, I've never wavered in my belief in humanity's ability—and our collective responsibility—to bring about a more just and equitable social order. I've always believed in humanity's potential to create a more caring society.

That viewpoint has infused my relations with family, friends, patients, and medical colleagues. It's been a lifelong, driving force to promote equality and the common good, and I believe it has served me well.

I suppose being a physician has made it easier for me to work toward this goal. Easier, that is, than if I had chosen a different occupation. I've spent a lifetime trying to help others—in my daily rounds, in my clinic, as a hospital administrator, at demonstrations, in my work with health advocacy groups—and it all adds up to a deeply rewarding career. Few people have such good fortune.

But as you've no doubt noticed in the preceding pages, my views and actions have also propelled me into sharp conflict with institutions and persons who would perpetuate injustice. That was true yesterday; it remains true today. My work is unfinished.

**

I look on my family—especially my children, stepchildren, their spouses, and my grandchildren—with great pride and love. I've been gratified by their many accomplishments and the extent to which their outlooks have been influenced by mine.

Three of my five children now live in the San Francisco Bay Area: Nancy, who worked for many years at a music production company; Polly, who practices family medicine; and Barbara, a psychotherapist. My son Ethan is a writer and editor in New York City, and my youngest son Michael is an academic librarian and professor of art history at the University of Connecticut.

It's a delight to spend time with all of them, their spouses and their children. (I now have nine grandchildren.) And of course I love my stepchildren, William and Karin Weaver, and their families, too. In fact, I practiced medicine with Stephanie, William's wife, for many years in Hyde Park.

**

As to whether I've seen social justice achieved in the public arena—in civil rights or in health care, for example—it's clear that despite some progress, we have much further as a nation to go. There is a widely propagated myth, for example, that in matters of race, "equality has been achieved." Similarly, there is an all-too-widespread myth that Obamacare and similar partial reforms will deliver "universal health care." Neither of these claims is true.

There have been important social advances in democracy, no question. The civil rights movement had a major and beneficial impact on every aspect of U.S. life. I was honored to have both witnessed and participated in this momentous battle for justice.

But here as elsewhere, much more remains to be done before full equality is achieved, and the gains of yesterday are subject to being taken away today or tomorrow. We need to redouble our efforts to extirpate racism from every aspect of the U.S. life.

We need to pass single-payer national health insurance, an improved Medicare for all. We cannot rest until everyone, without exception, has unimpeded access to high-quality care. We cannot accept "U.S. exceptionalism" in this department: with our resources, there is no justification for lagging behind any other country.

We need to radically reduce the huge wealth disparities in our country, where the vast majority of our economic assets are controlled by the "1 percent." We need to get big money out of politics and elections. And we need a more rational, humane foreign policy—and come to terms with the U.S. no longer being the overweening power in global politics. That's just for starters.

Over the years, I've been accused by right-wing circles of being "un-American" for having advocated for a more humane society. These charges have left me unfazed. I am merely an American who has exercised my constitutional rights. I remain unbowed.

Once I appeared before a congressional committee to testify in support of single-payer reform. One member of that august panel tried to provoke me by saying: "Dr. Young, what you're advocating for is free health care. If we were to go along with that, pretty soon people would be asking for free housing, free college education, free food, free transportation and more."

I replied: "Not necessarily, congressman. But I like your list."

**

I do take heart in my peers and in new generations of activists who are working for a more just society. Take, for example, The Albert Schweitzer Fellowship, a program that has inculcated (and continues to inculcate) large numbers of health-profession students with the highest values of socially conscious, altruistic medicine.

In the fullness of time, these students—many of whom will become tomorrow's physicians—will carry forward an earnest commitment to vanquish the many inequities in our health system. This pleases me.

**

Over my lifetime I've seen astonishing advances in science and medicine, including the the attainment of much greater sophistication and skill in the diagnosis and treatment of disease.

I've seen the average life expectancy rise from the mid-50s in the 1920s to the upper '70s today. These gains are indeed marvels.

Yet I've also seen how access to these medical achievements has been unevenly distributed. I've seen the stubborn persistence of dehumanizing inequality.

I've experienced some very dark chapters of history: the Great Depression, the rise of fascism in Europe, World War II, the Great Fear of the 1950s, and the threat of annihilation associated with the Cold War.

At the beginning of the 21st century, we have the material wherewithal for sustaining a large, healthy population and making new, dramatic advances in science, communication and culture —worldwide. But at the same time there is a rising capability of war and even planetary destruction.

To a certain extent this book chronicles, from a health viewpoint, the evolution of the tension between these two trends—toward justice or injustice—over the past century. Whichever trend prevails will define the 21st century.

I retain a terrible reputation for excessive optimism. The glories of humankind's ingenuity and inventiveness have not yet been exhausted. The future can be bright, but only if we work to make it so.

Glossary

AAAS—American Association for the Advancement of Science
AFSCME—American Federation of State, County and Municipal Employees
AIMS—Association of Interns and Medical Students
AMA—American Medical Association
AMSA—American Medical Students Association
APHA—American Public Health Association
ASTP—Army Specialized Training Program
ASU—American Student Union
BPP—Black Panther Party
CACOSH—Chicago Area Committee on Occupational Safety and Health
CCCO—Coordinating Council of Community Organizations
CEDCMI—Committee to End Discrimination in Chicago's Medical Institutions
Chicago 7
COFO—Council of Federated Organizations
COHO—Council of Health Organizations
CORE—Congress of Racial Equality
County/CCH—Cook County Hospital
GP—General Practitioner
HCA—Hospital Corporation of America
HHGC—Health and Hospitals Governing Commission
HMPRG—Health and Medicine Policy Research Group
HAS—House Staff Association
HUAC—House Un-American Activities Committee
LMD—Local Medical Doctor
MCHR—Medical Committee for Human Rights
MOBE—Mobilization Committee to End the War in Vietnam
NGO—Non-governmental Organization
NMA—National Medical Association

NU—Northwestern University

OEHO—Office for Equal Health Opportunity

OSHA—Occupational Safety and Health Administration

PNHP—Physicians for a National Health Program

PPC—Poor People's Campaign

RCP—Revolutionary Communist Party

SCLC—Southern Christian Leadership Council

SDS—Students for a Democratic Society

SEIU—Service Employees International Union

SNCC—Student Non-Violent Coordinating Committee

UAW—United Auto Workers

U of C—University of Chicago

UIC—University of Illinois at Chicago

UPP—Urban Preceptorship Program

CPSIA information can be obtained at www.ICGtesting.com
Printed in the USA
LVOW08s0305231013

358152LV00003B/4/P

9 780988 799660